PRAISE FOR
HEALTHY AS F*CK

"A no-BS guide to looking and feeling your best that doesn't make you want to cry into a salad? Hell yes! *Healthy as F*ck* is a different kind of weight-loss book—because it's not just about dropping pounds; it's about dropping judgment. Hilarious and legitimately inspiring. I loved it."

—Sarah Knight, *New York Times* bestselling author
of *Calm the F*ck Down*

"I love Oonagh's ability to cut through the crap and communicate simple, livable ways to eat healthy, exercise, and create new sustainable habits in a clear and direct way!"

—Harley Pasternak, international bestselling author
of *The Body Reset Diet*

"*Healthy as F*ck* is a smart, funny, and practical guide to revolutionizing your health and wellness. Oonagh Duncan addresses everything from mindset to meal prep in order to help you get healthy (and happy!) from the inside out. She'll make you laugh, she'll make you think, and she'll give you just the kick in the you-know-what that you need to put healthy habits into action."

—Ocean Robbins, bestselling author of *31-Day Food Revolution*

"Hilarious, laugh-out-loud funny, and straight to the point—Oonagh doesn't mince her words. If you want to get off the weight-loss roller coaster, ditch the exhausting diet mentality to feel and look your best, *Healthy as F*ck* is packed with advice that actually works because it's not about a diet; it's about a lifestyle."

—Joy McCarthy, holistic nutritionist and two-time bestselling author of *Joyous Health* and *Joyous Detox*

HEALTHY AS F*CK

The Habits You Need to Get Lean,
Stay Healthy, and **KICK ASS at LIFE**

OONAGH DUNCAN

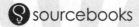

Dedicated to my parents, Susan McNerney and Bruce Duncan.

I truly won the life lottery to be born to two such incredible people,

and I'm so grateful for everything you've done for me. I love you

both so much. I'm sorry I swear so much in my book. x

Published by Sourcebooks
P.O. Box 4410, Naperville, Illinois 60567-4410
(630) 961-3900
sourcebooks.com

Library of Congress Cataloging-in-Publication Data is on file with the publisher.

Printed and bound in the United States of America.
MA 10 9 8 7 6 5 4 3 2 1

CONTENTS

PREFACE   v

PART 1: GET YOUR HEAD OUT OF YOUR ASS   1

INTRODUCTION: So, You Want to Lose Weight...   3

CHAPTER 1: Drop the Guilt and Get Your Hot Abs—
    Even If You Have a Women's Studies Degree   13

CHAPTER 2: Find the Fucks   22

CHAPTER 3: Woo-Woo Alert: It's Actually All about Happiness   38

PART 2: JUST TELL ME WHAT THE FUCK TO DO
    TO GET SKINNY ALREADY   57

INTRODUCTION: Why Discipline, Motivation,
    and Willpower Are Bullshit   59

CHAPTER 4: The Scoop on the Habit Loop   67

CHAPTER 5: The 7 Habits of Highly Healthy Motherfuckers   78

PART 3: HOW NOT TO BE A BIG,

    FAT QUITTY McQUITTERFACE   147

INTRODUCTION: Do. Or Do Not. There Is No Try.   149

CHAPTER 6: The Life-Changing, Magical Art

    of Getting Your Shit Together   153

CHAPTER 7: The Power of Your Peeps   174

CHAPTER 8: Break Up with Your Bullshit   188

CHAPTER 9: If You Can't Do Something Right,

    Do It Totally Half-Ass   208

CHAPTER 10: How to Fight the Fuckits   222

CONCLUSION   245

NOTES   248

ACKNOWLEDGMENTS   265

ABOUT THE AUTHOR   270

PREFACE

HAVE YOU EVER HEARD OF GLUTEN? IT'S THIS PROTEIN THAT'S found in wheat that...just kidding! It's the 2020s, and even your weird survivalist uncle is gluten free.

I bet you can name three people off the top of your head who would rather eat nuclear waste than gluten. That's why there are bestselling authors who could substitute the wheat flour in their baking with gold dust because they've made a fortune selling gluten-free cookbooks. Which is all kind of weird if you think about it...considering that celiac disease really only affects 1 percent of the population.

You know what else affects 1 percent of the population? Von Willebrand disease. It's this blood clotting disorder that probably none of your friends talk about at cocktail parties. Why? Von Willebrand disease isn't a covert way of pretending you aren't on a diet. Because

chances are you are on a diet right now. Except you don't call it a diet.
You call it a wheat allergy or eating clean or ketosis or paleo or plants
or maybe you are just trying to avoid sugar.

Now don't get mad. I know that accusing you of being on a diet is
like accusing you of being some vapid cheerleader who didn't get the
fucking fax in 1987 that diets don't work and you are supposed to love
yourself the way you are. You probably hate the word *diet* because
it reminds you of your mom counting her Weight Watchers points or
cooking nothing but cabbage soup for a week. Well, I'm afraid your
keto lifestyle might seem just as ridiculous to the next generation. And,
dude, I'm not judging you for getting super into the latest healthy-
food/weight-loss trend. We all follow trends. (Anyone else feather their
bangs in the '80s? Whoopsie daisy.) But let's face it—most people don't
really care if it's about sugar, wheat, free-range protein, or cleanse kits
with chlorophyll slime as long as there is a reason to hope it will help
trigger fat loss.

The point is, the language has changed, but as I type this, seventy-
five million Americans are *actively* trying to lose weight. Which is no
surprise. We are now at a point where *most* of us are overweight, and
more than 30 percent of North Americans are clinically obese. I'm not
talking about a little muffin top over your skinny jeans (although god
knows we are certainly made to feel like shit if this is the case). We are
at the point where we have to start thinking about type 2 diabetes,
heart disease, depression, cancer, and fertility problems.

So, the average American is freaking out and spending an average of $800 a year trying to fix the problem—buying juice cleanses, meal plans, workout programs, and weird-ass herbal supplements. And then everyone feels like shit about themselves. Why? Because none of it works.

I mean—obvi, right? The whole world is getting fatter. And the statistics of weight-loss success with any of these diets is dismal. And I mean *any of* them. Even that sugar-free thing you're doing right now. From Atkins to the Zone with a lot of keto and GF in between—there is no peer-reviewed scientific data that confirms that one diet (or—excuse me—"lifestyle") is better than any other for long-term weight loss. There is very little chance—across the board—of keeping the weight off for over a year.

Here's why: it's not about your wheat intake, your ketones, or your net carbs—*it's about your habits.* The National Weight Control Registry at Brown University studies those rare unicorns who have lost significant weight and kept it off. They achieved it through all sorts of different diet/lifestyle approaches. The research shows that the *one* commonality in those subjects was making small changes to their everyday behaviors.

Small changes to everyday behaviors?! How fucking *boring* is that? Where is the "revolutionary new formula"? The "one secret that doctors don't want you to know"? Or the "diet that celebrities swear by"?

That is all Satan's bullshit.

Let me tell you, if you like sensationalist clickbait headlines, this book is going to disappoint. On the other hand, if you like having an effortlessly healthy (smokin' hot) body and a calm mind, welcome to your new life.

I call those "everyday behaviors" your habits. Everything comes down to habits. All the rest of it—everything from the glycemic index to complex intermittent fasting protocols—all of that is just noise and fad diets disguised as a virtuous lifestyle.

Now before you hit send on that angry email where you tell me that getting rid of gluten has changed your life and how dare I call it a diet: I'm happy for you. If you've found something that works for you, then you can shut this book. You don't need my advice because you've already got this shit nailed—and that is awesome. Celebratory rice cakes all around!

But.

If that gluten-free "lifestyle" tends to fall off when you are stressed or when there's something particularly delicious in front of you or when you are on vacation...that is a diet.

Consider this: When is the last time you heard a vegan say that things were so crazy at work that she was gonna give herself a break and eat meat until life calms down? Or hearing someone say that they were going to pause their tooth-brushing habit while they were on vacation because, you know, you only live once! Ridiculous, right? Because veganism and tooth-brushing are deeply ingrained habits. They are part of your identity. They require no perceived extra effort because they are rooted in a deep sense of the kind of person you are. ("I just don't eat meat. Period." Or "I am someone who does not have nasty-ass teeth and fart breath no matter how relaxed and on vacation I am.") So, unless your sugar-free/gluten-free/paleo/keto efforts are completely effortless and it never occurs to you to pause them on vacation, you are on a diet.

And so what if you are? There's nothing wrong or shallow or unenlightened about wanting to lose weight (more about that in chapter 1), so props to you for trying stuff out. The only reason I'm taking a big second-day-of-the-Master-Cleanse dump all over your "lifestyle" choice is because it's not going to be sustainable and it's going to end up making you feel like shit when it doesn't work out. Again.

And I say fuck that. I never want you to have that yucky, "I totally fell off the wagon, I suck" feeling again. That's why I wrote this book. That cycle of getting your hopes up with a new weight-loss program and then feeling like a loser when it fails? That shit is over, my friend.

I'm talking about that weight-loss roller coaster. You know, where you try this new thing (coconut oil all over everything! net carbs be damned!) that has a bunch of pseudoscience to back it up and omigod it totally works and you announce to everyone that this is IT, you are totally doing this now, and it's not a diet it's a lifestyle, but then one weekend you just don't fucking feel like doing that lifestyle but whatever, you'll pick it up on Monday and then Monday rolls around and you pick it up but it's kind of lost its joy but you dutifully do it because this is totally your thing now but then Wednesday is your friend's birthday and a girl's gotta celebrate good times come on, so then Thursday doesn't count because you are hungover and then it's the weekend so… Yeah.

You'll probably futz around like that for a few months or so and you'll have moments when you pat yourself on the back for being "good," but those moments will probably start to get fewer and farther between...and then the Fuckits will take over (more about the Fuckits later), and then in a year, you'll probably slide back to where you started. But maybe at that point you will be excited for the next roller coaster. Maybe it's all about probiotics now.

It's not that all those fad diets/lifestyle experiments are evil or stupid or anything. The problem is that they are a costly distraction from what is actually going to help you reach your goals: your habits.

Think about it. We all know what to do. Eating vegetables is not a secret. The benefits of exercise aren't exactly breaking news. Most of us have figured out that water is a healthier choice than a Wildberry Cooler. It's not that we don't know what to do. We just don't know how to make ourselves do it. Consistently. Automatically.

In this book, I'm inviting you to get off that roller coaster of highs ("I'm really doing it now! This is totally my thing!") to lows ("I suck. I'll never be a fit person and I should probably just accept it."). Instead, I want you to come ride the merry-go-round of healthy, repeatable habits. A merry-go-round where you basically repeat the same stuff day in and day out. There are highs and lows, but it's just the horse bobbing up and down gently—nothing you're going to lose your lunch over. The merry-go-round is way less exciting, I know. There are no "secrets" or "ground-breaking techniques" that will blow your mind. You won't have that high when all you can talk about are ketones and how you've found the next big thing. Instead of the thrill (and crash) of the roller coaster, the merry-go-round is generally pleasant, but it doesn't take all your attention. It just keeps going around. You will probably lose interest after a while.

Which is fucking awesome.

I don't know about you, but I've got better things to think about than weighing my food or calculating the calories I burned during a spin class. When you are taking care of your health intuitively and automatically, you can save your precious brain power for shit like running for office, closing the gender wage gap...or just enjoying a damn meal with your family without worrying about "being good" or "following rules." Let me tell you—eating without all that bullshit is so much more delicious.

And that's what I want for you—a delicious quality of life in every way. Because of the healthy habits I'm about to teach you in this book, I now have a body that I'm thrilled with. And not in a fakey-fakey, "I love my tummy because it's a reminder of the fact that my body carried two beautiful kids" type of way but in a "who wants to see a million pictures of me in my bikini?" type of way. But the real gift is a brain that is completely uncluttered with thoughts about "how to lose belly fat fast." It's fucking *rad*.

I certainly didn't start out this way. If you told my twenty-year-old self that I would become a fitness expert, I would have tripped over my platform boots and dropped my cigarette. I am not one of those fitness professionals who came out of the womb doing cartwheels and swinging a shiny ponytail through life. More of a participation ribbon kind of kid. While other kids were running around the schoolyard, I would have been hiding in a bathroom stall reading *Harriet the Spy*.

As I blossomed into womanhood, I decided that I liked beer, Whoppers with extra mayo, and guys who wore capes and eyeliner (but that's another story). Point being that by the time I hit my late twenties, I was sedentary, puffy, and unhealthy. I felt uncomfortable every time I sat down because my waistband cut into my belly. I'd always be picking my shirt away from me so people wouldn't see my rolls. There was no way I'd wear a bathing suit in front of my friends, no matter how inviting the pool looked. In group photos, I'd always go to the back and try to hide half of my body behind someone else. I was always bigger than my boyfriends in an era where "waif" and "heroin chic" were what was considered hot. (I mean, WTF, right?!)

I know what some of you are thinking: *Cry me some first-world tears.* I'm not saying my life was a Greek tragedy or anything; I've never been obese or faced the kind of discrimination and health problems that obese people face. But I was always thinking: *If only if I could lose ten, twenty pounds, everything would be so much better.* Whenever I'd schedule an upcoming event, I would start to scheme about how I could lose ten pounds before the big day.

So, I tried all these things (familiar, anyone?):

- I tracked my food.
- I ate low fat.

- I did yoga.
- I had meal replacement shakes.
- I didn't eat past 8:00 p.m.
- I skipped breakfast.
- I drank nothing but lemon water with cayenne and maple syrup for ten days.
- I tried diuretic teas to release (*ahem*) "water weight."
- I made cabbage soup.
- I ran a half marathon.
- I ate nothing but salad.
- I ate nothing but meat and butter and cream because carbs were bad.

And year after year, I got fatter.

Not only fatter, but I was exhausted from all the effort. Worst of all, I was unhappy with my body and mad at myself for not being able to just lose the weight. So I drank too much wine and smoked too many cigarettes. Every time I saw a picture of myself I thought, *That can't be me.* It was impossible that I was that girl in the mirror. And I was so *pissed* at myself for not being able to nip it in the bud. I was smart and generally accomplished... Why wasn't I able to make myself *do* this?! I would punish myself for "being undisciplined" by skipping meals or doing longer workouts. I signed up for a really expensive gym membership with orange slices and fancy lotions in the change rooms because I thought that if it was really expensive that would force me to go and get my money's worth. (It didn't, by the way. I walked in, felt like the only person there who wasn't already in amazing shape, tried to get a machine to work, and didn't know what I was doing. Walked out. That visit cost me $300.)

So it wasn't that I wasn't trying. I was trying really hard. And I bet you've tried really hard. It is not your fault if this shit hasn't worked. It's nothing to be ashamed of if you've been caught up in the weight-loss roller coaster. Most importantly, don't you go hatin' on yourself if you think about this stuff too much and you think you should be above it all.

The weight-loss industry marketing cycle is a powerful force that is worth $66 billion. (That's a *B*, y'all. We are talking serious coin here.) And all that weight-loss hype is making us all fatter (and sadder). But the good news is that by picking up this book, you are politely excusing yourself from that $66 billion party and instead have already started making a huge shift toward developing healthy habits, mental freedom, and a totally slammin' body.

Imagine this: You wake up with tons of energy. Probably didn't even need the alarm clock. You easily slip into clothes you love and you are totally happy with what you see in the mirror. You spend the day feeling energized, clear-headed, and positive. You can eat anything you want but you automatically choose the healthy food that makes you feel good and satisfied and you never ride that wave between starving and stuffed. The ripple effect of your healthy habits has been fantastic. You are in a better mood for your family, you have more confidence at work. You feel kind of sexy for the first time in about fifteen years and the effect on your relationship has been…um…how shall we say… fucking hot. Not only that, but your whole family has started to shift their habits along with you. Your kids are better behaved, and your husband has more energy and seems younger. (*Ahem.* See above re: relationship.) You've got a little extra money in your pocket because you aren't flushing it down the toilet on expensive supplements (literally…you think your pee is naturally that color?). Best of all—you've got all this extra time and brain space that you used to spend tracking your macros and trying to burn off extra calories at the gym. Now you can spend that time hanging out with your girlfriends, starting a business, saving the whales, or whatever the fuck you want to do with your life.

Here's how it's going to go down: In part 1, I'm going to encourage you to "Get Your Head Out of Your Ass." This is the mindset stuff you are going to want to skip, but let me say this in very clear terms: DON'T FUCKING SKIP IT. Otherwise, you are screwed. We are going to get totally clear on why you want to lose weight in the first place. (Newsflash: Maybe you actually, um, don't want to lose weight. Maybe this project doesn't even need to happen. #mindblown.)

Then we are going to make sure you understand that it's actually a feeling you are chasing—not a number on the scale. You don't really care about losing twenty pounds—you care about having the feeling you think you will have when you lose twenty pounds. Maybe you want to feel sexy, or strong, or confident... In any case, that shit is only going to happen if you start practicing that feeling now—at exactly the weight you are at. You heard me. It's Law of Attraction time: if you want to feel good, you've got to focus on feeling good. Roll your eyes if you want, but if you skip this stuff, you are doomed to repeat your old patterns. Just telling you now.

Part 2 is "Just Tell Me What the Fuck to Do to Get Skinny Already," and this is where we get down to the nitty-gritty of why you haven't been able to sustain any healthy living initiative so far and why this time is going to be different. Expect some smarty-pants research that you can quote at dinner parties if you insist on being that asshole. Then we are going to get into the 7 Habits of Highly Healthy Motherfuckers, so you can stop getting distracted by clickbait bullshit and instead focus on eating your vegetables like a grown-ass woman.

Once you've got your healthy habits down, I'm going to teach you in part 3 "How Not to Be a Big, Fat Quitty McQuitterface." We'll get super-practical about designing your environment in "The Life-Changing, Magical Art of Getting Your Shit Together" and then get really deep in your self-sabotaging mental muck in the final chapter, "How to Fight the Fuckits." You know, those moments where you think, *Fuckit, I'll start on Monday*? I've got a solution for that.

Ready to make this the last time you start a healthy living project? Because it's time to reclaim your brilliant brain, your bangin' body, and your delicious life. It's time to get Healthy as Fuck.

. PART 1 .

GET YOUR HEAD
OUT OF YOUR ASS

SO, YOU WANT TO LOSE WEIGHT...

SO. YOU WANT TO LOSE WEIGHT.

That's not even a question—it's pretty much a given these days. There is the assumption that if you don't have a freaking thigh gap, then you should want one. And you are kiiiiiind of lazy if you aren't working on it.

Don't get me wrong. As a society we *are* kind of lazy. We move too little. We eat too much crap. There are rising rates of obesity and type 2 diabetes in children, fer fuck's sake. But somewhere in between—

I can't see my feet/an entire season of Game of Thrones *is my idea of a marathon/yes please I would like that super-sized.*

And

Washboard abs/ultramarathon running/eating an entire banana is my idea of a wild night

—there is a lot of room for *being normal*. Which is totally healthy.

So just pause for a second and think: What if you decided that you didn't have to lose weight after all?

I know. It's crazy. Just stay with me here.

I know you want to be healthy. If you didn't, you wouldn't have picked up this book. (And if you are seriously out of shape, uncomfortable, facing health issues, and your habits are such that you barely managed to take your hand out of the KFC bucket to open this book, then I am so excited to help you change all that. No judgment. I got you, girl.) But what if you are more in the muffin-top category? The "I've been trying to lose the last ten pounds for the last ten years" category? The truth is that your belly fat is probably totally normal. And healthy. (If you want to double-check, I've got a quick assessment at www.fitfeelsgood.com/book.)

I'm guessing you don't like the way it *looks*. That's totally fair. (And in the next chapter, I'll go on to explain why there is nothing shallow or unfeminist about wanting to get fit just because you think it looks hot.) But before you decide to change your habits in the name of hotness (as you will learn to do in this book), it's worth considering that the body ideal you are striving for is probably just a fashion trend that is exaggerated by highly processed and Photoshopped images. Fashions change and so does the ideal body. Imagine if people had subjected themselves to shoulder implants to conform to the shoulder pad rage of the 1980s. Trying to attain a certain look that happens to be popular right now might not be worth the pain in the ass—or the abs. Even if the coveted thigh gap (or whatever is the latest thing) could be realistically achieved, it's totally possible that a different body type will soon be in favor.

Even in my tender young lifetime (*cough* forty-two years *cough*), body trends have varied wildly. I can remember times when Kim Kardashian's bum would have been an embarrassment. I clearly remember distinct periods of wanting to look:

- diminutive (but top heavy) like Winona Ryder in *Reality Bites*
- gaunt and vulnerable like Kate Moss for Calvin Klein
- powerful and badass like Linda Hamilton in *The Terminator*

By the time we all manage to "break the internet" with champagne glasses balanced on our prominent Kardashian butts, the pendulum will swing back toward Twiggy again and we'll all start freaking out about having defined collarbones or something and be incredulous that we ever worried about our butts at all.

The truth is that body trends are as transient and fickle as the butterfly collar or the overplucked eyebrows of the '90s that we all deeply regret. There's nothing wrong with following trends or wanting to look a certain way—I still freaking *love* that Linda Hamilton look—but you've got to make sure it's worth it before you drag yourself through another "Let's get fit now, seriously this time" effort.

Look down at your body right now. Seriously—do it. (Extra credit:

Try to do it with love and no judgment.) These are the simple facts: the body you are looking at right now is the result of:

1. Your genetics
2. Your habits

It's as simple as that.

You can't choose your genetics (obvi). But you can absolutely choose your habits and therefore change your body. Which is what this book is about. And in consciously choosing and creating your habits (rather than defaulting to your norm) you are consciously choosing the body that is right for you. It might not be the body that society thinks you should have. It might not be the body that you had once for about fifteen minutes at the peak of doing some completely unsustainable diet. It *will* be the body that is the result of your genetics and your *chosen* habits that you can cultivate and sustain for life. The habits that actually make you feel good.

Because here's the deal: It's not that hard for most people to move from having an unhealthy amount of body fat to having a healthy body composition. But it might be a serious pain in the ass to go from a normal amount of fat to being super "cut," depending on your genetics. The great news is that *you* get to choose. Not society or fashion trends. In fact, you must choose. Or you will be fucking miserable.

Let me give you an example. My awesome and hilarious friend,

Beth, was obese for most of her life. Her parents were big, and she grew up in a household with unhealthy habits—lots of TV and most dinners were takeout or frozen microwave meals. In her twenties, she decided to stop drinking Coke all day and start walking to school and back. In doing so, she dropped a lot of weight, and although she was still chubby, she could shop at "normal" clothes stores, and she felt much better. She got so many compliments, and she was really happy with her success.

Beth was easily able to maintain her new habits, and her weight normalized at her new set point. After a while, everyone got used to her new weight and stopped mentioning it. Beth noticed that the compliments had dried up and worried if she still looked good. She decided to kick it up a notch, and she went on a strict low-carb diet (even picking the croutons out of her salad). In doing so, the compliments returned, and Beth was able to get down to a weight that she had never dreamed of. She did it. She was one of the "skinny girls."

But.

She was also kind of fucking miserable. She had to really plan out her food before going anywhere, and it was a pain in the ass. She had gone from being the "fun, outgoing one, who was up for anything" to the one who never accepted a bite of your dessert and anxiously asked the waiter whether there was any sugar in the glaze on the salmon filet. In short—she was at her dream weight. But she found it fucking HARD.

Here is an example of an effort-to-results graph for Beth:

BETH'S GRAPH

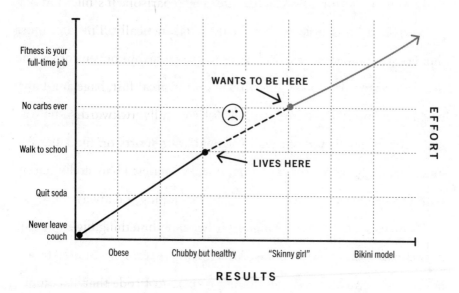

So, I'm guessing you know what happened next. Beth couldn't sustain her extreme low-carb diet and she reverted back to what was a more natural set point for her: no Coke, daily walking, dessert occasionally, eating the shit out of the croutons on the salad. And, given her genetics, this meant she was no longer "one of the skinny girls."

And I wish I could report that Beth made this choice consciously and is totally at peace with it, but instead, she's like most women in modern society. She starts every week weighing herself and feeling like a failure because she's not at that goal weight she was once. She tells herself, "That's *it*! No more croutons! No more dessert—you can have flavored soda water. It's time to get back to being one of the skinny girls. For real this time." She gives it a shot for a day or two and of course, it proves to be too hard to sustain for long. And so the cycle continues.

It doesn't have to be this way.

Let me tell you another story as a comparison. It's mine. As I've mentioned, I was always a bit chubby. Genetically, I'm lucky—my parents are both lean—but I grew up with the carby convenience habits of a lot of kids in the '70s and '80s: cereal for breakfast, bagel for lunch, pasta for dinner. I was also extremely physically awkward and would have preferred to die than be caught playing sports or, like, "trying" at something. By the time I'd reached my twenties, I had slowly gained enough weight that when I'd go clothes shopping, I'd always reach for the very back of the rack and hope there was something big enough to fit me, even though I'm only five foot four.

I tried everything to lose my belly fat, and I rode that weight-loss roller coaster like I had a season's pass and I wanted to get my money's worth. Eventually I developed one of the 7 Habits of Highly Healthy Motherfuckers that you are about to learn: exercising consistently. In doing so, I got quite a bit fitter, and I was reaching toward the middle of the rack when I went clothes shopping. Maybe sporting a muscle or two. But when I nailed down my nutrition (again, using the habits you are about to learn), that's when my body really started to change. I'd go into a clothing store and the saleswoman would hand me a pair of jeans to try on and I'd look at her incredulously, thinking she'd mistaken me for a twelve-year-old.

And I know that sounds like a happy ending, but, like Beth, I found this "peak skinny" hard to maintain. It required that I measure all my food and avoid any alcohol. Drink my coffee black. I was doing it, but the austerity didn't quite match my sense of who I was.

So I decided to consciously choose a different spot on my graph.

Did you catch that? I made a choice. I didn't "fall off the wagon"; I consciously decided that fitting into the tiny teenager jeans wasn't worth the effort. This is where I think my story deviates from Beth's and from so many other women, who are constantly beating themselves up in the quest for perfection. Instead of relentlessly striving for peak skinny and berating myself for not adhering 100 percent to the strict rules that made it possible, I have decided to love the body that I have when I'm eating well 80 percent of the time. Because that feels like a reasonable effort to me. You might like more freedom than me and want to put less effort into your healthy lifestyle. Or maybe you are happy to be totally hard-core and eat well 90 percent of the time.

The point is to choose your effort consciously—and then your only job is just to be happy with the results. I never look down at my belly (and yes, I have a belly) and think, "Dammit! Why did I screw up at that restaurant when I was out with my friends and have drinks and appetizers?!"

Instead, I look down at my belly and think, *This is the belly I get when I choose to eat well 80 percent of the time. I chose this belly. I could choose to have a six-pack, but that would mean that I would track every calorie and never have a glass of wine. I already know that is not the right choice for me. It makes me less happy. I also know that if I were to eat healthy only 50 percent of the time, my belly would get bigger and I'd feel sluggish and that would make me unhappy. THIS is exactly the belly I have chosen. Now I get to love it.*

The problem, I think, is that most women operate like Beth. Constantly striving for a body that doesn't match the effort that they can give sustainably. And they are constantly beating themselves up about it—rather than just letting that "ideal weight" idea go fuck itself.

So, what if:

- Your body fat is not that unhealthy and totally within the range of normal?
- The specific body type you desire—whether it's a tiny waist, huge shoulders, a big bum, or a thigh gap—is probably just an unrealistic fashion trend that's likely to go away in a couple of years?
- Getting leaner would be possible...but maybe not worth the effort?

Would you still want to lose weight?

What if...as of this moment...you were no longer hoping to lose a couple of pounds? (I know it's crazy, but stay with me here.)

What kind of space would that free up in your life?

- Would it create room for other meaningful self-improvement projects? What intellectual or spiritual pursuits might be fun to explore if you were finished worrying about what your belly looks like?
- Would you stop punishing yourself with exercise and start participating in movement that you love?

• Would you start focusing on other health metrics—sleep, stress reduction, and maintaining positive social connections?

I'm not trying to dissuade you from wanting to lose weight. On the contrary—my transformation from a chubby, inactive person to someone of above-average fitness who freaking can't wait for bathing suit season has been one of the most rewarding journeys of my life. The ripple effect into every area of my life has been incredible. I'm so excited to share it with you so that you can recreate a life-changing transformation in your own life.

But I want you to start this transformation understanding that *YOU get to decide on* the body you want. And it may be the body you currently have. Or, it may be that you will choose a body with six-pack abs.

Either way, your journey to loving the shit out of your body starts now.

· CHAPTER 1 ·

DROP THE GUILT AND GET YOUR HOT ABS—EVEN IF YOU HAVE A WOMEN'S STUDIES DEGREE

ONCE UPON A TIME I WAS A FAT ACTIVIST. WHICH IS NOT AN activist who happens to be chubby (although I was that too). A Fat Activist is someone who advocates to change anti-fat attitudes in society. And now I'm a fitness expert who is writing a book about how to lose your fat.

I'm telling you this story because I want to invite you to drop any first-world guilt you might have about wanting to lose your muffin top—and give you total permission to go and be the MILFiest MOFO you want to be.

My activist journey started in 1998, when I was front-row center in my Women's Studies 101 class. Doc boots were ON. The prof put up a projection of this ad from the Body Shop that had a graphic of a chubby Barbie doll with the caption: *There are three billion women who don't look like supermodels and only eight who do.*

It's the kind of thing that people would share on Facebook today and everyone would heart the shit out of it.

The prof asked for our reactions to the ad and you might be surprised to hear we tore it to shreds, but it was a Women's Studies class; that is what you *do*. The prevailing objection to the ad was that the Body Shop was supposedly promoting self-love while profiting from our insecurities by selling us products. If we didn't all want to look like supermodels, then why would we want to buy your peppermint foot cream? This led to a discussion of how The Man is keeping us enslaved by perpetuating such a narrow definition of beauty that we spend most of our lives being distracted by chasing that ideal instead of smashing the patriarchy.

Fast-forward a couple of years and I became a full-on Fat Activist while on tour with a musical theater company. For a year I traveled with a cast of about one hundred singers and dancers in what was basically a petri dish for eating disorders. For example, people would get a part in the show on the condition that they lose a certain amount of weight before the tour started. When we showed up for duty, we were all warned that if we gained weight during the tour, we might lose our role because "you will no longer fit into the costume." To make matters ickier, during the show, management would have chubby people with beautiful voices singing backstage while thin people lip-synced into dead mics onstage. Not only that—we were given no control over our food choices during the tour, which was provided by the company. Cue bulimia epidemic, stage right.

Fresh from my Women's Studies days at university, a few renegade castmates and I staged a revolt. We advocated for "body-blind" casting and wrote letters to the management to insist they rewrite their policies. Within our cast, we attempted to neutralize the word *fat* as a body tissue, not a pejorative. We talked about how obesity is socially constructed and not a personal failing of character or commitment to one's health. We taught that big can be beautiful and that people with lots of body fat are not automatically unattractive, lazy, or unhealthy.

And I still believe all these things. *With all my heart.* I never assume that a person with extra body fat wants to lose weight. I never assume that someone eating a Big Mac combo doesn't know what they're doing. I never compliment someone on having lost weight like that's invariably a good thing.

This is where my mindset was at when I started my fitness company, a company that came as a bit of a surprise. I had started teaching exercise classes after my tour because it was enough like musical theater to satisfy my needs: colorful spandex costumes, cheesy music, everyone looking at *me*—so it met many of my late-twenties essential job criteria. Even though I felt like a little bit of a fitness impostor (it's possible I might have had a smoke on my way home from class once or twice during those early transition years), teaching exercise classes helped pay the bills while I wrote and produced documentary plays that were supposed to change the world. After some minor theatrical successes, I had a sudden epiphany that I actually liked teaching my fitness classes more than my theater stuff. A bunch of my clients gathered together and asked me to start a boot camp, and that's how I found myself one day standing in a park at 6:00 a.m. with a bullhorn wearing a T-shirt with my new company name on the back.

But you see, mine was a *different* kind of fitness company! I called it Fit Feels Good, and we were all about feeling good! We never talked about weight loss! We never posted before-and-after pictures or talked about getting your body ready for summer. But in doing all of this, I was *completely* ignoring a major reason why my clients were hiring me. The truth was that most of my clients wanted to lose weight. As I type these words, more than half of American women are trying to lose weight. And in my insistence on a "feel good," health-oriented-only narrative, I was effectively silencing them. And I was judging their deepest desires. And I didn't even realize it.

Then I met the Orange People and I changed my mind. You know who I'm talking about. Those people who do bikini or bodybuilding competitions. They live in the grunting section of the gym, get an orange tan, and then flex onstage in a crystal bikini with a blinding, neon smile and a butt harder than marble? The Orange People were those for whom I would have reserved my snottiest eye rolls during my fat activism days. As such, they were not people I would have met through my social scene. But at this point in my fitness career, I was training and certifying new personal trainers, many of whom were bodybuilders who wanted to pass on their knowledge. And guess what? Umm...they were really knowledgeable.

Sculpting a specific kind of physique and timing it to be in peak aesthetic shape on a specific day takes some serious scientific chops. It also takes a hell of a lot of work. My (admittedly lovely) bodybuilding students would proudly show me their competition photos and I would gasp at the extent of their transformation. (Because, let me be totally clear: They never looked like that in person. That fitness-magazine-cover glory is a one-day event. Totally impossible to sustain. But I'll pass on some useful information from the Orange People in later chapters because it's crazy interesting stuff.) And so I grudgingly started leaking some admiration toward those Orange People.

And then I began to wonder why their event, the one they trained so diligently for, was any different from any other peak athletic event that we all generally accept as a worthy pursuit. Was it really so much more admirable to run a marathon than to compete in a bikini show? Both require extremely hard training and self-discipline. Neither activity particularly benefits society. Okay, sure, maybe you collected a couple of bucks for the charity run, but let's be honest, that was a bit of an afterthought. I think we can all agree that most people are doing it for themselves and for the sense of accomplishment it provides them.

Which is fucking GREAT.

Can you imagine what would happen if more women just did shit for themselves and for the sense of accomplishment? I don't care what it is. Walk the West Coast Trail. Drop ten pounds and fit into a size 6. If you're squashing those aspirations because you think they're shallow or selfish, you're doing yourself—and society—a huge disservice. And women do squash their aspirations. All the time. Let's take a look at a typical conversation between two women, one of whom wants to lose weight:

> **Jen:** "I'm on a diet! I want to lose ten pounds so I can look like a smokin'-hot MILF at my son's bar mitzvah next month!"
>
> **Michelle:** "What? That's *ridiculous*! You don't need to go on a diet! You're perfectly fine the way you are!"

At a glance, this looks like a perfectly acceptable exchange. Jen's ambition isn't particularly noble or anything. She doesn't need to lose weight for her health. She just wants to look hot. And Michelle is just being a good friend by telling her that she doesn't have to change a thing. My problem with it is that Michelle is (a) stating her opinion about Jen's body, which is kind of irrelevant, and (b) squashing Jen's ambition.

Imagine if we played that game with women who want to make more money.

> **Jen:** "I'm starting a side business! I want to make $100,000 a year so I can treat myself to sweet-ass vacations!"
>
> **Michelle:** "What? That's *ridiculous*! You don't need a side business! You have a totally average income and your vacations are fine the way they are!"

Obviously that would be a total bullshit response that completely disrespects Jen's ambition and her right to say what she wants for her own fucking vacations.

To expand on the income analogy: I'm not saying that everyone needs a high income. Just like I'm not saying that everyone needs a magazine-cover body. It is perfectly possible to be happy with an average income, and obviously money isn't everything. It is also perfectly possible to be happy with an average body, and looks aren't everything. But if you *want* to make a gazillion dollars and have Tina Turner's legs, then You. Fucking. Go. Girl. Don't let anyone squash your ambition and mansplain to you that "you need to love yourself the way you are."

There's nothing self-loving about resigning yourself to a body that you aren't proud of, that doesn't feel good, that doesn't reflect who you want to be in the world. There's nothing shallow or selfish about wanting to be the absolute best version of yourself, whatever YOU decide that is. In fact, it's the greatest gift you can give to the world. And yet, the idea persists that getting rid of your muffin top is a shallow or selfish pursuit, and that taking care of everybody else first is what makes a woman noble.

> There's nothing self-loving about resigning yourself to a body that you aren't proud of, that doesn't feel good, that doesn't reflect who you want to be in the world.

Right now my primary mission is running my online transformation program. And I can't tell you how often I'm asked this question when someone is thinking of joining: "Will my family like this food?" Not "Will I like this food?" Not "Will these foods help me feel good from the inside out?"

The irony here is that taking care of yourself, focusing on your dreams, your health, and your ambitions actually does end up being good for the whole family. Because when Mom gets fit, the whole family gets fit. When Mom gets healthy, she's modeling healthy habits for everyone. And when Mom is happy and feels confident in her own skin, she radiates. And the whole world benefits.

Here's the truth: People register for my online program in order to lose weight. And they do, don't get me wrong: twelve pounds on average. But then guess what happens when those women find themselves residing in a body that feels good to them? When they've built the confidence that comes with setting a hard goal and doing the work to achieve it? Guess what happens when they create solid habits that eliminate the need to spend precious brain bytes counting calories and carbs?

> Wanting to get leaner, stronger, sexy AF isn't the patriarchy getting you down. Feeling shitty about your body is the patriarchy getting you down.

A *lot* of stuff happens.

When Denise finally dropped below the two-hundred-pound mark after years of struggle, she realized that it's possible to change her life in any way she wanted, and she decided to start an online business. Michelle got the confidence to start dating again. Diane lost thirty pounds, got off her diabetes medication, and felt amazing when walking the red carpet at her play's Broadway opening. Lisa lost only ten pounds before she got the courage to quit her shit job and move to her dream cabin in the mountains. Wanting to get leaner, stronger, sexy AF isn't the patriarchy getting you down. Feeling shitty about your body is the patriarchy getting you down.

This is *your* life. So don't you dare feel guilty or shallow or unfeminist about wanting to lose your muffin top or sculpting your Kardashian butt or whatever you want to do with your own damn body.

The ultimate act of defiance is to love your body *right now* exactly as it is and then shoot for the stars to make it the most badass Temple of Awesome that *you choose* it to be. If that means a six-minute mile, great. If that means six-pack abs, great. If that means being a bit orange and turning sideways while flexing, great. Our job as woke women is to accept every *body* exactly as it is without judgment (including our own) and to cheer on anyone who is working to improve themselves— whatever that means for them.

· CHAPTER 2 ·

FIND THE FUCKS

I'VE GOT GOOD NEWS AND BAD NEWS.

The good news: getting lean and healthy and staying that way for life is actually pretty simple. The bad news: if you want different results than you're getting now, you're going to have to do something different.

You would think that's a big "Um...duh." But, let me tell you, if there's one thing that people hate, it's changing their behavior. I mean, a lot of people will tell you that they are an easygoing, go-with-the-flow type person, until you ask them to go with a different flow than the one they are used to.

Take the hundreds of people who pay good money for my online transformation program. Usually they will have heard about the program from a friend who got great results, or maybe they read some review online. In the beginning, they are so excited to get lean and healthy once and for all that they're practically doing jumping jacks in front of their computer. They slap down the investment, thinking this time it's going to be different.

Then they get their grocery lists and menu. They show up in the Facebook group asking if it's okay to adjust the program to accommodate their current habits. "Can I still have toast with peanut butter every morning? Because I really love my toast with peanut butter."

At this point I have to gently ask if their current habits are giving them the results that they want. The disturbingly obvious answer is no. Which totally sucks for them. Because most people are pretty attached to what they are currently doing. To admit that what they are currently doing doesn't work would be to say that they had wasted all that time and effort. It would be like admitting you just spent the past ten years digging for gold and then learning that there was never any gold in them thar hills. You had been given the wrong map. Usually, by the time they get to me, they have been digging for a long time.

Imagine you run half marathons and do yoga and eat a low-carb diet. You've been doing that for so long now that it's part of your identity as a fit person. But the truth is that you aren't seeing the fat loss results you want. What's your natural, totally understandable response? You run more and do more yoga and start eating beef jerky for breakfast and try to kick-start some results around here. But you get more frustrated because you're noticing diminishing returns from all those efforts. The routine that used to work well isn't delivering the same results, and you are busting your ass just to maintain your fitness, and nothing is improving no matter how hard you try. You start to think: *How much more diligent must I be? How much harder must I work? Is something wrong with my thyroid? Why does God hate me?*

The truth is that when it comes to weight loss, most people are executing Einstein's definition of insanity: doing the same thing and expecting different results. Is it any wonder that so many people feel batshit crazy when it comes to weight loss?

I know you might be working hard already and putting in a solid effort. You might already be logging your hours on the treadmill and ordering the salad dressing on the side and Googling sugar-free, grain-free muffin recipes. But if you aren't getting the results you want, I'll say that that effort is good for only one reason—it satisfies a puritanical work ethic of being industrious and busy. I'm going to argue that you are actually letting yourself off with "easy effort."

What do I mean by easy effort?

It's a concept that's made the rounds in personal development circles, but I heard it from John Berardi of Precision Nutrition. Easy effort is hard work that feels familiar. Kind of like putting in time at a job you hate. Or playing the martyr in your family by doing all the housework. Putting up with bullshit in your marriage in order to avoid having a confrontation. Taking another online course on how to be a life coach instead of just putting yourself out there and doing it. Running three miles a day because it's what you've always done. All that shit is hard work, but it's the devil you know. It doesn't require a lot of mental effort. It also requires nothing new from you. It allows you to feel busy but ultimately will never really change anything.

> Real effort frightens the bejesus out of you. Easy effort is just a slog you have to get through.
> Real effort demands improvement. Easy effort lets you stay basically the same.
> Real effort accomplishes something meaningful. Easy effort lets you tick a box on a to-do list.

Change happens when you drop all that distracting busywork and actually try something new. You know, the stuff you've been avoiding because it's too intense? The stuff you probably suck at because you haven't put the required practice time in yet? The stuff you can't manage while you're in autopilot mode so you make yourself too busy so you have a good excuse not to try it? Yeah, that stuff. That's the stuff that would put you on a whole new trajectory.

That's what I'm talking about.

I'm going to ask you to suspend all your "rules of healthy living" that you may have accumulated through years of various diets. It may feel uncomfortable or even scary AF. Instead, we're going to get back to basics and create healthy habits that will last for life.

The act of building new habits and skills will require some effort. You're going to have to use your brain when you don't want to. You'll have to unplug from autopilot. You'll need to surrender to being sucky at new skills for a little bit. You may have to deal with a little grumping from the people around you who liked things the way they were. But if you want to change your body, you have to do something different. And yes—doing something different can feel hard. But the good news is this: those healthy habits are eventually going to be effortless. (I'll tell you how soon, so chill.)

Think of anytime you learned a new skill and what a pain in the ass it was when you first started. Think back to that first week at your current job. The new procedures, the names you had to remember, the skills you had to develop. It probably felt a little overwhelming. While I was trying to get my acting career off the ground, I worked briefly as a travel agent. And at the end of those early days at my travel agency I felt like my head was going to explode trying to learn all the computer codes to pull up the fares for the various airlines and then add on our commission and taxes, etc., etc. I'd flop onto my couch at the end of the day with a shaking hand holding a glass of pinot grigio and sob into the phone to my best friend, "I can't do it! I swear to god, travel agents are the smartest people in the world."

While I still hold the utmost respect for the intelligence of travel consultants, I will say that I eventually got the hang of it and it didn't seem like that big a deal. I could quote fares while doodling on a piece of paper and wondering what was going to happen on *Ally McBeal* that night.

The same thing will happen with your Healthy as Fuck journey.

At the beginning, it's going to feel like a lot of work. Your first BBQ without beer might feel like agony. Your first day without five cups of coffee might feel like moving through ectoplasm. The first time you don't "help" your child finish her ice cream cone might feel like everything is wrong in the world. But you can do it. And after a while it will become absolutely effortless. And just because it's effortless doesn't mean bullshit easy effort. I'm talking about foundational skills that deliver continuous results. But you'll only get there if you want the results badly enough.

You know who the real badasses are when it comes to pushing through the really hard stuff? Who don't fuck around with bullshit effort but constantly make the kind of effort that's actually worth a damn? Little kids.

The other day I was watching my six-year-old son at skating lessons. He would glide a few feet before his feet slipped out from underneath

> When was the last time you pushed yourself through that level of pain in the ass in order to build a new skill?

him, sending him sprawling onto the ice with zero dignity intact. With minimal drama, he got back up and did it again. And again. And this was the effort-cherry on top of a day at school where he struggled and stammered through every word as he learned how to read. That's working hard for real.

When was the last time you pushed yourself through that level of pain in the ass in order to build a new skill? Because most of us adults will give a little effort and then give up, saying that we "don't have the time right now" or "life is too crazy." It's usually crazy with busywork. It's up to you to clear space and energy for the important shit.

It's understandable: Humans are like any other living organism. We seek pleasure and avoid pain. Which is why every now and then I'll have a client who says, "I want to lose weight, but I just can't stop eating cheese and drinking wine every night!" I'll respond, "If that's the case, then you don't really want to lose weight."

I'm not saying that to be a total bitch. I'm just pointing out that she clearly associates more pleasure with cheese and wine than getting in shape. The problem is, she *thinks* that she wants to lose weight. But in the moment, she *feels* like wine and cheese. And guess what? Your feels are going to win over your brain. Every time.

Did I just tell your life story? Don't freak out. Girl, I *got* you. We are breaking that cycle now. And remember—I told you that I currently eat healthy about 80 percent of the time. This isn't about forbidding wine and treats for the rest of your life. I don't want to live that way, and I'm guessing you don't want to either. This is about creating automatic healthy habits that allow for those exceptions with minimal impact. When you have automatic daily habits that serve your goals, you can also have a habit of a small Friday-night indulgence and still have a body that is getting fitter. But if you can't seem to get those consistent daily habits off the ground and you are stuck in a pattern where you just can't execute the behaviors that you know you should, I guarantee it's because you associate more pain with changing your current habits than the pleasures of what is on the other side of that change.

That's why I'm not just shoving a bunch of workouts and recipes at you. This is where we collect all the Fs—all the fucks and all the feels—that are going to drive you forward, over the hump of changing your current behavior so you can create healthy habits for life.

This is where we find your *why*. Because if you're going to choose unsexy delayed gratification over the ever-so-alluring immediate variety, we're going to have to switch a few things up. We're going to have to create some strong new associations.

Ready? As we move through the next section I want you to actually stop reading, close your eyes, and really reflect on this stuff. Even better if you write this stuff down. If you aren't a "Dear Diary" kind of person, I get that you might feel like a doofus, but let me tell you something—it's a lot more doofus-y to spend your whole life wondering why you can't make lasting behavioral change. When you take a moment to close your eyes, feel this shit, and actually write it down, you get mad props for real effort, rather than the easy effort of skimming the page.

First, I want you to connect with the pain of your current situation. WARNING: THIS WILL SUCK. That's the point. I want you to go *there* and inject all the feeling you can into it. You know all those feelings and insecurities that you drown in food and booze and distraction and fake news? Yeah. We are going to feel those now. Put on your big-girl panties.

Write down what will happen if things stay exactly the same as they are right now, if you continue on your current trajectory. For example:

If nothing changes, I'm going to continue to get heavier every year. I will spend the rest of my life feeling uncomfortable every time I sit down because my waistband is cutting into my belly. I will always feel a little out of breath. I will always worry that my kids and my spouse are embarrassed to introduce me to their friends. I will spend every summer feeling sweaty and uncomfortable because I don't want to wear shorts and a tank top. I will start to get health issues that will seriously impact my enjoyment of life and worry my family. I will never have the energy to do the things that I want to do.

Do you feel seriously yucky yet?

If not, go back and re-do it. Remember—you will naturally avoid pain and move toward pleasure. We need you to feel the pain of your current situation, or you won't have enough fucks to fix it. Write that shit down in a rainbow diary with a lock if you need to, but do the work.

Now I want you to close your eyes again and take yourself to pleasure island.

You know the hopes and dreams that you don't allow yourself to really connect to because you've tried losing weight so many times that you can't bear to get your hopes up again and it's easier to believe there is just something incurably wrong with your adrenals or your big bones or your genetics? *GO THERE.* What will life be like if you *nail* this thing? What would be so freaking *awesome* about having exactly the body and energy that you want? What if you were actually the hottest person you know? What would you do with the extra brain space if you never thought about losing weight again? What would you do? What would you wear? How would you feel? For example:

If I had the body and health of my dreams, my entire life would be fucking amazing. I would wear such awesome outfits and I would feel proud about the way I look. I'd walk out of the house thinking, I hope I run into ALL my exes at the grocery store today. I would be that fun mom who has the energy to run around laughing and playing with the kids and I could just let loose with them and I wouldn't feel like a fool or out of breath. They would love it so much if I actually climbed on the playground equipment and chased after them. I'd have so much more energy to get shit done that I'd basically be superwoman checking shit off my to-do list like no one's business. Garage organized? Book club started? Cat taken to the vet? Check, check, and check, bitches. I could stop being tired all the time and be in a much better mood for my family. We'd fight so much less and actually enjoy each other's company. And don't even get me started on what it would do for my relationship if I started feeling sexier and initiating some midweek lovin'. I might even buy some undies that aren't entirely practical and give my partner a heart attack. And then I'd strut into work with so much confidence (in my awesome outfit) that my boss would be like, "Wha? Who is this amazingly brilliant leader and why has she been hiding behind her computer all this time?" Basically—I'd be the person I was always meant to be. I could stop hiding my awesome.

You should keep writing until you feel like you are going to burst with excitement about your hot new bod and your new, amazing, healthy life. You should be mentally picking out bikinis with a big-old smile on your face. You should feel so pumped up about your vibrant health that you want to run out of your house and arm wrestle unsuspecting strangers just so they can feel your POWER. Your new goal should feel not only exciting but absolutely essential.

Keep going until you feel connected to your deepest sense of self and what's important to you. Remember that the difference between going on a diet or trying something for a while and actually changing your life for real is changing your sense of identity. You need to distill your "why" down to the core of your new identity. You've got to OWN this shit.

I want you to finish the end of this sentence: "I am going to push through the initial discomfort of habit change and lose weight once and for all because I am the type of person who..."

For example:

...lives life to its fullest and there's no way my physicality is going to get in the way of that.

...models healthy living for my kids and brings my best self to all my relationships.

...will not tolerate being sick, boring, and tired. I have one life to life, and I want it to be awesome.

Keep going until you feel like you are going to cry when you read your one sentence about the kind of person you really are and why you are going to lose the weight once and for all. This is your "why." These are your *F*s.

Now I want you to stay with *that* feeling. That feeling, that identity that you've just connected to—that's the person who is going to skip the wine and cheese. *That* person doesn't give a *fuck* what's on Netflix at 11:00 p.m. because they have a workout to get to the next morning. That is the person who is going to push through and actually have the balls to make real change, who won't get distracted or placate themselves with easy effort that is actually just avoidance of the real shit.

Once you've found your *F*s, I want you to hold that vision and ignore everything else. I mean it. Don't let any obstacle steal your attention. It's all about that vision.

Now, I know this sounds like your standard goal-setting vision board shit. But let me tell you about how I saw this work in real life. It happened while I was pretending to die an excruciating death in theater school.

The acting exercise seemed simple: We were told to imagine that we were in a room—and we had to leave the room in absolute silence or we would die. It was up to us actors to come up with some imaginative circumstances around this premise, but the most important part was doing the emotional preparation for the scene. We had to imagine how we would die and really connect to what was at stake—the potential pain, the consequences of getting it wrong. (*Ahem.* Just as I've encouraged you to do just now.) In this case, you have to picture actors huddling in all corners of the room, listening to death sounds on their headphones for proper gruesome inspiration. People were looking at pictures of their family that they wouldn't see again if they made a sound while trying to get out of the room. I burned a little pile of my own hair and smelled it to imagine my flesh burning. Like, we WENT there.

The next part of our emotional preparation was to focus on the objective: why we wanted to live. Which we sort of fuffed off a bit because, like, who doesn't want to live. Duhhh. Also, we were theater students and it was much more dramatic to wallow in the hair burning, etc.

What happened was this: One by one, we all failed the exercise because we made a noise while trying to escape and therefore "died." Sometimes the actor would scuff the carpet a bit, or their knee would crack as they stood up. But always, *always*, because the door to exit the room creaked. I mean the motherfucker CREAKED. There was no way around it. And every time, the prof would raise his eyebrow, shrug, and say, "You're dead," then mark a big, fat *F* next to our name in his notes.

Eventually we all started to get pissed and protested that the assignment was ridiculous. The fucking door CREAKED. There was no way to escape the room silently! It was physically impossible. To which my unsympathetic prof replied, "If you want to live, the door will not creak." I thought he was a total dick.

Until someone passed the exercise.

I still remember it. Her name was Christine. She was calm from the very start. (Most of us were quivering wrecks by the time we had done our "emotional preparation" for the scene.) She had unwavering focus on the door. When she started to move, there was no question of her joints making a noise—she was floating across the room. Every movement was fluid, economical, and purposeful. She reached that fucking creaky-ass motherfucking door that had been our collective undoing for weeks (causing untold actor hissy fits) and put both her hands on it and slowly, confidently, opened it and escaped.

It was the most beautiful and fascinating thing I had ever seen. We were all gobsmacked.

"That," my prof said with a steely gaze at the class, "is what happens when you truly want to live."

Unlike the rest of us drama queens, Christine had spent less time mentally jerking off on grisly imaginations of her own death and instead got Absolutely Fucking Clear on why she was going to live.

And this is how you need to be about your new body and health. It's happening. You are going to make it happen. You are going to be like my son who never asked to quit skating lessons even though he bailed on his face all the time. Because he's a little boy growing up in Canada. Giving up on skating would be like giving up on walking. It's just not an option. You are going to be like a little kid learning to read, no matter how frustrating it is to build that skill because reading is fucking rad and there's no way you are going to grow up illiterate. That's what it feels like when your objective is part of your identity, when it's rooted in your deepest values.

Look, I know you skipped that exercise above when I told you to find your *F*s. When I asked you to really go there and find that statement where you distill all those amazing feelings of why this life change is important to you down to one essential sentence about your identity. But I'm telling you that if you don't find the *F*s right now, this journey is going to be a short one. You are going to skip to part 2 and take a stab at "the diet," and then two weeks later you are going to come down with a case of the Fuckits. And I suspect you've already tried that strategy.

I repeat: Weight loss is actually really simple. There's actually a chance that you will have to do LESS in order to release the last ten pounds, twenty pounds, or whatever you are working on. But in order to get different results you are going to have to do something different.

Shifting your habits is going to challenge you. And I mean *really* challenge you—not just add more easy work that makes you feel like you've checked a box. If you are going to rise to meet that challenge, you are going to need a strong reason why. So if you didn't do the exercise, I suggest you go back and do it now.

Once you are all fired up and so fucking clear on why you are going to live—I mean *really* live, in a body that feels amazing to you—let's just skip to the good part and get you there immediately. Like, now.

CHAPTER 3

WOO-WOO ALERT: IT'S ACTUALLY ALL ABOUT HAPPINESS

IF YOU ARE A FELLOW CHILD OF THE '70S OR '80S, YOU MIGHT remember a *Sesame Street* book called *The Monster at the End of This Book*. The story revolves around Grover, who is freaking out because he heard there is a monster at the end of the book. As you turn the pages with your grubby toddler fingers, he gets more and more frantic, with illustrations of him trying to nail the pages together to avoid getting to the end and facing the monster. And, of course, when you get to the end, the monster is him. Cute, adorable, lovable Grover.

It's some deep shit if you think about it.

This may not be what you want to hear, but I'm just gonna go ahead and say that this book ends the same way. Your weight-loss journey ends the same way. Even when you achieve the body of your dreams, there you are. The monster is you. If you have a lack of confidence now, that same lack of confidence will creep in, even at your goal weight. After the initial rush is over, your brain will find its default settings, and no matter how hot you look in those jeans, you are going to feel pretty much the same way you do now.

And this is where you say, "*What?* That's bullshit! If I've done all the work to get down to my goal weight, I want to feel like Scarlett Johansson!"

Exactly—you want to *feel* like Scarlett Johansson. You don't actually want to lose weight. Let's get clear about that. Do you really care about your gravitational pull on the earth? Nah, fuck the earth—you just want to be buff. Why do you want to be buff? Because you want the feeling you think you will have when you are buff. Sexy. Confident. Free. Proud. Happy.

It's the *feeling* that we really want—not the actual weight loss.

This is one of the most misunderstood things about goals: we usually lose sight of what we truly want. We think we want that sweet job or a million bucks or for George Clooney to give us a massage. But no, we want the feelings we think will ensue—in essence, happiness.

Don't believe me? Think about it. Take any goal you have and ask yourself *why* enough times, and you will always get to *happiness*.

Example: I want to win the lottery.
Why? So I can buy a geothermal biodome and live in the country.
Why? So that I can feel in harmony with nature and hang out with
    my family.
Why do you want to do that? Because it will make me happy.

Example: I want to have visible abs.

Why? Because I want to rock a bikini with pride.

Why? Because I'll feel sexy and proud of myself for doing
   something really hard.

Why do you want that? Because it will make me happy.

Do you see what I'm getting at? You don't really care about having a flat belly or qualifying for the Boston Marathon or whatever. You care about *feeling* gorgeous, athletic, energized, alive, attractive, light, accomplished. Basically, happy.

What I'm proposing is that you skip right to the end and start working on being happier NOW. Otherwise you are going to get to the end of the book and discover the monster of unhappiness is right there waiting for you—at any weight. You'll get your flat abs, but then find that your upper arms are utterly unsatisfactory. And that is not a cute surprise like it was for Grover at the end of the book. Your lack of fulfillment will ultimately create a monster that will set you up for a lifetime of discontent. There is no way I'm going to let you get to the end of this book and find that monster. That Monster of Dissatisfaction can totally suck it. Starting now.

Which is why we are going to start the most important part of your training program immediately—and that's training your brain to access those happy feelings. Right now. At exactly the weight you're at.

Here's the thing, my love: if you can't be happy now—at exactly the weight you're at today—you won't be happy at your goal weight. It will be like trying to use a muscle that has atrophied from lack of use. Just like you've got to train your upper body muscles so you can do push-ups, you've got to train your brain to be able to access your sexiness, your confidence, your freedom, your pride, and your happiness.

Now I can practically hear some of you shouting at me: "But, Oonagh, I can't practice feeling happy now—you don't understand. I'm, like, *gross*. I've got this secret cellulite that no one knows about, and my thighs chafe when I walk out of the shower, and my boobs rest on my belly when I sit down, and if anyone ever saw me naked with the lights on they would turn to stone..." Etc., etc.

First of all, I hate to take away your special snowflake identity, but everything you think is secret and gross about your body is probably totally common and normal. We just never see it.

Side note: This is why I kind of think everyone should be naked all the time. It would be the ultimate smackdown to the shame that so many people have about their *totally normal* bodies.

When I was traveling with that theater company, one of the coolest things we did was tour Scandinavia and stay with local families. Taking a sauna is a part of basic hygiene in Finland, so my host family would often ask if I needed a snack, a drink, or a sauna. Coming from Canada, where a sauna is a fancy-schmancy spa thing, I opted for the sauna when the opportunity first presented itself.

So there I am, sitting in this wooden box with my towel wrapped around me, congratulating myself because the steam is probably good for my pores or something, when much to my horror, the whole Finnish family comes in to join me—*whipping off their towels* to sit on them, and casually asking if I have any brothers or sisters back at home.

I later grilled my Finnish friend (FF) about this shocking mixed-gender family nudity:

Me: "So, you've seen your dad...naked?!"

FF (laughing): "Of course! He's my dad! You've never seen your dad naked?"

Me (barfing): "Of course not!! He's my *dad*!"

For us, growing up in North America, nudity = sexy times. So, the only nudity we see is in porn (or ads and Instagram feeds that are trying desperately to look like porn). Finnish kids grow up seeing normal body diversity in their peers and parents, and there are studies that indicate it leads to a much healthier body image later on in life. I know my two boys are going to be exposed to my post-breastfeeding boobs until they weep for mercy. And when they get older and realize that nudity actually does = sexy times occasionally, they will be going into those situations with realistic expectations about what human bodies actually look like.

So, whenever you feel shame or embarrassment about your body, know that what you think is hideous and unlovable about your body is probably totally normal and on display at a Finnish sauna somewhere at that very moment.

Second, I'm going to challenge you that it is totally possible for you to be happy or sexy or whatever you want to feel at exactly the weight you are right now. Let's look for evidence that this is possible.

Have you ever seen anyone who is your size or larger who is sexy? I just Googled "sexy plus-size celebrity," and now this book is never getting written because I'm just gonna stare at Danielle Brooks and Ashley Graham all day. If it's possible for them to be gloriously hot at their size, why not you at your size?

On the other hand, can you collect any evidence that skinnier doesn't always equal sexier? Have you ever seen anyone who is skinnier than you but holy-shit-not-sexy-at-all? I'm thinking about Mr. Burns from *The Simpsons* as my Exhibit A.

The point here is to bust your false beliefs that your weight is what determines your sexiness. Keep researching until you are forced to admit that it's *possible* to be as fat as you are right now and still be sexy as all hell. And that even when someone gets skinnier it doesn't always mean they're sexier. Once you've got overwhelming evidence of diverse bodies also being hot as hell, I'm hoping you might realize that even *you*, with your hideous, probably-totally-normal-and-therefore-glorious body can be sexy and happy right now, at exactly the weight you are. Once you believe it's possible, it's time to start training. Because if you want to feel sexier when you lose weight, you've got to start accessing that feeling *now*.

Throw on your "Eye of the Tiger" confidence mix. (If you don't have a playlist of sick tunes that make you feel like strutting, go to my site and grab mine: www.fitfeelsgood.com/book.) Bust out the clothes that make you feel incredible at exactly the size you are right now. Dance in your living room. Sing sultry torch songs in the car on the way to Walmart. Wear red lipstick to vacuum the house. Go flex in the mirror and congratulate yourself on being A Powerhouse That's Not to Be Trifled With. Take your first belfie (butt selfie) and send it to someone who deserves to bask in your magnificence.

And yeah, it might feel like total bullshit at first. But that's no different from any muscle you are trying to train. When you first start working out, you are weak as hell. Because you've never asked your body to do anything, your body has wisely conserved the energy and allowed those muscles to atrophy. You also haven't created any neural pathways to do that particular motion, so it feels super awkward.

Then, you start doing push-ups. Your body will say, "Holy shit! Girl is doing push-ups! We need to figure this out neurologically and also strengthen those muscles, so we suck less and get the job done."

The same process applies to feeling sexy, confident, and happy. When you first start practicing these feelings, you will feel awkward and weak, but the only way to get better at it is to train and start practicing. Because, again, the ultimate goal is those feelings.

On the other hand, if you've been training for something your whole life, you will be amazing at it. Let's say you were a trained belly dancer. You would automatically start twitching your hips when music comes on. You wouldn't even have to think about it. Your core muscles would be strong because you would be used to activating those muscles. You would also feel totally confident in a belly top because, like the physical act of dancing, feeling confident and sexy in a belly top is a neural pattern you'd been practicing your whole life. No big whoop.

The problem is that most people who want to lose weight have been practicing shitty neural pathways of discontent and self-hatred. They are literally training themselves to feel shitty by repeating their negative thoughts over and over again. For example, if you look in the mirror every day and think, *Gross. I hate my muffin top. I look like someone stuffed Jabba the Hut into skinny jeans. Look how it hangs over my pants. I need to cover that shit up. I would be so happy if I didn't have a muffin top*, then here's what I can guarantee you: You won't be happy when the muffin top goes. Because you haven't been practicing being happy. You've never looked in the mirror and found something positive to think. Your brain hasn't built those neural pathways. How could it even know where to begin thinking positive thoughts? It would be like expecting your muscles to do a full pull-up when you've never even carried your own groceries.

If you continue to focus on negative thoughts and somehow managed to lose your muffin top, you will look at your new body in the mirror and think, *I'll be happy when my thighs don't touch.* Or *Look at all that gross, loose skin. I should look into surgery.*

And here's the other thing—you probably *won't* lose your muffin top if you are looking in the mirror and thinking, *Ugh, I hate my muffin top.* It will probably just get bigger.

Because that kind of self-hating bullshit *doesn't work*. It has the opposite effect.

A 2017 study from McGill University found that feelings of shame and self-criticism are associated with increased hunger and weight gain. On the other hand, feelings of confidence helped with habit regulation and weight loss. Another study done at Duke University asked women to eat doughnuts quickly. After the doughnuts, some of the women were given messages of self-compassion, telling them not to be hard on themselves for indulging. The other half didn't get any self-love message. Later on, the women were given bowls of candy and invited to eat as much as they wanted. Guess who ate almost three times as much candy? The ones who didn't get the reassurances that it was okay to eat the doughnut.

I know you think that if you play boot-camp sergeant with yourself, you will be able to shame yourself into behaving properly, but negative, self-hating thoughts will lead to negative, self-hating behavior. There is no other outcome. No one ever *hated* themselves into a body they loved. That has never happened.

Remember the pleasure and pain exercise from the last chapter? I had you connect to the emotional pain of your current trajectory in order to change it. But once you've got that emotional fuel, you've got to be 100 percent focused on what you want: the pleasure of having the hot and healthy body you want. Remember the story about the one girl in my theater-school class who focused on her objective of living versus the rest of us who kept focusing on why we didn't want to die? She was the only one that lived. Let me give you a few examples of how this self-love-positive-thinking-woo-woo shit plays out in the real world when a girl is just looking to lose a couple of pounds.

Example 1: My client Cathy had a beach vacation planned, and it was important to her to look and feel amazing for her big trip. The problem was, she really didn't. She hadn't been on top of her food and nutrition for the past couple of months, and she was feeling it. So, she posted in one of my online groups: "Okay guys, I'm going to try a cleanse this week to get in shape for my trip—wish me luck!"

A few days later she posted: "So much for my cleanse. I just killed a bunch of toast with half a jar of peanut butter. What is wrong with me? I can't believe how much I suck."

Now imagine these two alternate versions for Cathy's inner get-ready-for-vacation monologue:

Cathy #1: "Oh shit, shit, I screwed up so badly! I can't believe I'm so fat. I've got my trip coming up! How did I let this happen? I suck!"

Cathy #2: "Even though I'm not at my goal weight yet, I still totally love myself and the body I'm in right now. I'm going to have the best time on my trip. I'm going to make mostly healthy choices with a few indulgences and come back feeling refreshed and ready to smash my fitness goals. I'm so excited for ALL of it!"

Cathy Number 1 is mad and disgusted with herself and feels like she should be punished. Cathy Number 2 is realistic about her body's current condition but still giving herself tons of love, with full confidence and excitement that she is on her way to achieving her goals. Now you tell me, who is going to have more fun on her trip? Who is going to come home and end up getting ripped and healthy? And who is going to end up in the peanut butter again?

Example 2: You are going to a wedding. Your ex will be there. For whatever reason, you've gained fifteen pounds. It's time to put on your dress and it's, um…tight. Like, two sizes too small.

Internal Monologue #1: "SHIT! Fuckfuckfuckfuck this is too small omg I can't believe I'm so fucking FAT! How did this happen?! It's all those cookies from that bakery on the way home from work. I can't believe I'm such an idiot. Well, what am I going to do now? Everyone is going to be talking about how fat I am. Maybe if I wear a blazer over the top, people won't notice. But I will get heatstroke in a blazer. Well, that's the price I pay for allowing myself to get into this condition. That's it. Right after this wedding weekend, I'm going on a cleanse, and I'm never eating those cookies again, and I'm only going to have salad all this week. This sucks."

Internal Monologue #2: "Whoa! This dress is tighter than I remember. Well, I guess that's what happens when you discover an awesome new bakery that's on the way home from work… WHOOPSIE DAISY. But actually, it kind of looks sexy in a Kardashian-over-the-top kind of way, and my boobs look AMAZING. I should remember to lean over all the time to show off—this is by far the best cleavage I've ever had. And my legs look amazing in heels. Why don't I wear heels more often? Could I be that mom who does the grocery shopping in heels?"

Now, which one of these people is going to have a wicked time at the wedding and be super attractive? Which one is going to end up looking tense and weird and probably cry when the bouquet hits her in the face? Which one is probably going to drop the extra fifteen pounds over the next few months? And which one is going to start a cycle of "cookies to cleansing" and wind up even heavier?

Now, don't freak out and think you are doomed if you are someone who currently has a pattern of negative thoughts. Next time you catch yourself having harsh thoughts, here is your new pattern interrupter: *Even though I sometimes beat myself up, I accept myself exactly as I am. Besides, the fact that I am now aware of these negative thoughts means that I'm getting sick of this script and it's time to move on. Yay, me!*

Example 3: I got this question from a client named Tina. "What is the best way to burn more body fat, especially on the front and back of thighs? I eat mostly well, feel very strong, and I'm working out, but how do I get defined muscles and reduce the appearance of cellulite on my thighs?"

I know Tina personally. She isn't lying when she says that she eats well and works hard and has muscle…and she probably isn't lying when she says she also has cellulite. (About 90 percent of women do. If Tina lived in Finland, she would know this and wouldn't expect her thighs to look like marble.)

So, as a personal trainer, I was faced with a decision. My first option: I could tell Tina about a whole bunch of strength-training exercises that will build her quadriceps and hamstrings. Tell her to limit her already healthy eating and reduce all carbs and alcohol to really lean out and get some definition. Tell her about using Preparation H and fake tanning cream to reduce the appearance of cellulite. (Little tip I learned from some of my bodybuilding students when I was teaching the Personal Trainer certification course. Told you those Orange People know their shit.)

So yeah, Tina could achieve her goal, but it would be a lot of work. And I suspect that Tina has enough work to do in her life. Putting in that kind of effort for her thighs would probably be way beyond the effort that Tina could sustainably give. Here's an example of an effort-to-result chart for Tina:

TINA'S GRAPH

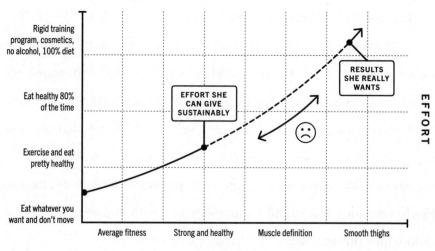

My other option was to ask Tina WHY she wants muscle definition and no cellulite on her thighs.

She'd probably roll her eyes and say "Duh," but if I asked her "Why?" enough times, we'd probably get down to the fact that she wants to tone up her legs and reduce the appearance of cellulite to feel confident and hot in a bathing suit or short shorts.

And who would blame her? Feeling confident and hot RULES. But I would argue that the most efficient way to achieve the goal of feeling confident and hot is simply to practice feeling confident and hot with the thighs you have. Like I said, confidence is the first muscle you need to train.

So here was my suggested training program for Tina:

- Do activities, listen to music, and wear clothes that put you in the state of feeling confident and hot.
- Hang out with people who think that you (and your thighs) are fucking awesome. Ghost on anyone who makes you feel yucky about yourself.
- Challenge yourself to go ahead and wear the short shorts, and every time you hear yourself thinking *Oh no—can they see my cellulite?* try to replace that thought with something like *Everyone is looking at my hella hot legs. You're WELCOME, world.*

Now, I'm not saying this stuff is easy. But on the other hand, neither is a grueling leg-training program combined with no carbs or alcohol. And which one will make you happier in the end?

Here's *my* example of training my confidence and happiness muscle. I have always been self-conscious of my midsection and wanted to challenge myself to bare my midriff with confidence. This is a picture I posted on Instagram right before making my shirtless debut at the gym:

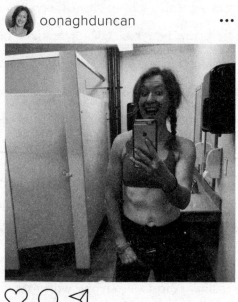

oonaghduncan   ...

131 likes

Now, some of you are probably thinking, *Easy for her to practice feeling confident—she is skinny!*

And others might be thinking, *Huh. Her body isn't that hot. I don't know if I would go topless if I were her. Yikes.*

And some of you may be thinking, *Jesus—did she really post that? I can totally see her nipple.*

And to all those thoughts I have two things to say:

1. As I mentioned, I breastfed two kids. Nipples happen. (Finland knows what's up.)

2. What other people might think about my body is their shit. I have no control over it. I'd go bonkers if I tried to antic- ipate what people might think of my body and adjust it accordingly. And it's not my responsibility. I have one—and only one—responsibility, and that's *my* shit. And by "shit" I mean my thoughts and feelings about my body.

Those thoughts and feelings about my body are the exact muscle that I was working on that day at the gym when I decided to expose my never-seen-before, pale-ass midriff and walk around the gym like some kind of glorious glowworm.

And here's what I did to control my shit for my shirtless debut (about which I was minorly terrified, which is why I had to have that pep talk with myself in the bathroom) and strengthen my feelings of confi- dence: anytime I caught a glimpse of myself in the mirror, or heard any of the usual self-criticizing mental chatter, I gave myself a completely outrageous compliment. *They should really start paying me to have a membership here, showing up looking this good.* Or *I look so hot that people are probably hoping I don't wipe down the equipment after I use it.*

Feel free to get ridiculous here. The point is not to delude yourself into believing that you can quit your job to start a modeling career, but to interrupt your pattern with humor and start to build positive associations with your body. Those outrageous compliments made me giggle a bit internally and, yes, made me happier and more confident.

Now, does this mean that we just go around doing whatever the fuck we want and as long as we keep the vibes high, we will lose weight and be happy? Not quite. Often when you ask people what would make them happy, the answer involves a corkscrew and a Netflix binge. This is an example of confusing happiness with pleasure.

Here's the difference: Pleasure is a momentary feeling that comes from some external source. The external source could be circumstantial (you just made a sale, that hottie texted you back, you found an awesome parking spot, you got the job) or sensual (you just ate something delicious or tucked into a cozy bed on a cold night). Happiness, on the other hand, is internal and long lasting. It's the difference between the *pleasure* you feel when someone gives you a compliment ("You look like you've lost weight!") versus the *happiness* of feeling so good in your own skin that you don't give a fuck what other people think of your body.

Pleasure is hitting the snooze button on a cold morning. Happiness is feeling yourself getting fitter and stronger and healthier from your morning workouts. Pleasure is sleeping with the hot stripper at your friend's bachelorette party. Happiness is playing footsies with your farty, but very funny, partner.

Now, I'm not knocking pleasure. Pleasure is a very good thing, and too many people are depriving themselves of pleasure for no good reason. I think people should give and get as much pleasure as they can out of life. The problem arises when pleasure comes at the cost of happiness. In order to have happiness, you have to feel like you are progressing toward your goals in a meaningful way.

So if you are looking for pleasure at the end of a fork or the bottom of a glass, it's time to quit it and find something else that's going to make you feel good in the moment. And I have suggestions coming up for that in part 2. We are about to get super practical on how to apply all this woo-woo shit.

But before we get there, I want to commend you for actually taking the time to Get Your Head Out of Your Ass. There are a whole bunch of people who are going to skip ahead to part 2: "Just Tell Me What the Fuck to Do to Get Skinny Already." They are in danger of approaching this

The problem arises when pleasure comes at the cost of happiness.

whole thing like just another diet. They are looking for the book equivalent of the meal replacement shake system.

You are the one who took the time to go deep and get clear on why this weight-loss stuff can be such a head fuck. In doing so, you have a much better chance at building healthy, long-term habits that are gonna make you one healthy and lean, sexy motherfucker.

Before we continue, let's review what you've figured out so far:

1. Do you actually want to lose weight? Is this a priority for you right now? If you do, that's totally awesome, and don't let anyone try to make you feel guilty about it!

2. Do you give enough *F*s that you will change your habits, even though you might be pretty damn attached to your current habits?

3. Do you understand that it's not really weight loss you want, but the FEELING you think you will have when you lose the weight? And that you need to practice accessing that feeling right now, at exactly the weight you are?

Check, check, check, and check? Awesome. Let's do this.

PART 2

JUST TELL ME WHAT THE FUCK TO DO TO GET SKINNY ALREADY

· INTRODUCTION ·

WHY DISCIPLINE, MOTIVATION, AND WILLPOWER ARE BULLSHIT

WELL DONE, YOUNG GRASSHOPPER. YOU HAVE COMPLETED THE essential step of getting your head out of your ass when it comes to weight loss. Now, let's get down to the nitty-gritty. This is like the part in *The Karate Kid* when Mr. Miyagi finally teaches Danielsan how to do some freaking karate, after he's been waxing the damn car all summer.

Are you ready for me to unleash the New Revolutionary Secret to Long-Term Weight Loss, Vibrant Health, and Everlasting Happiness (patent pending)?

Drum rollllllllllllll…

Eat your vegetables.

Get enough exercise.

Get enough sleep.

Wait a second. Why did you just throw this book across the room? Are you telling me you already knew that?! Well, duh. You've always known exactly what you need to do to get healthy. And I don't even mean in a fucking Yoda "the answer lies within" kind of way. I mean there was probably a poster in your kindergarten classroom that broke that gripping health-and-wellness story.

It's not that we don't know what to do. We need to admit that we just don't know how to make ourselves DO IT consistently for the long term. Remember how I mentioned that behavior change is hard?

Check it out:

- Twenty-five percent of people abandon their New Year's resolutions after just one week.
- An overwhelming 60 percent of people have bailed on their resolution by February.
- The average person will make the same damn resolution five times without success.

And it's not that people don't want to change! I know people who would rather lose weight than be sent on an around-the-world cruise with John Stamos. (That's everyone else's fantasy too, right?) But they still can't make themselves stick to it. It's not that they aren't motivated. Motivation has nothing to do with it. Studies show that even after a heart attack, only 14 percent of patients make any lasting changes around eating or exercise.

What the hell is going on? Are we just the most disgusting, weak-willed life-forms who can't get our shit together, even though our very lives might depend on it? Nope. But we are going about it all ass backward. We try:

Discipline: Strict rules about what we can and can't do/eat/ drink. We vilify certain food groups or eating after 8:00 p.m. or whatever the current trend is.

Motivation: We make a Fitspo Pinterest board, we sign up for an expensive gym, and we make a bet with our friend that we'll have to donate to the Men Who Have Perms Foundation if we eat a pie.

Willpower: We force ourselves to get out of bed and work out, and we give ourselves harsh talks in the mirror. We swear to all that is holy that we will NOT try that new hipster artisanal hot dog place that just opened up. Nope. Not happening. Not even if it damn well kills us.

But here is the problem with self-discipline, motivation, and willpower: they take a lot out of you. All those rules and mental shenanigans? That is a major life suck. Oh sure, it might feel kind of fun at first...like when you first decide that you are going sugar free and you rip your cupboards open and purge all the evil sugar that lies within and triumphantly post on Instagram about it, and the first few times you get to announce your new sugar-free status to all your friends and how good you are feeling.

Then fast-forward six weeks when you are stuck in traffic on a hot day, hangry and stressed with a screaming baby in the back seat, and the only food in the car is a box of Girl Scout cookies. Chances are you are going to be all outta *F*s for that whole sugar-free thing.

The truth is that we have better things to do than make Being Sugar Free our new full-time job, so as soon as the rush is over and something else happens that requires your attention and energy (say, I don't know...work, kids, living your GD life), you won't have anything left to execute your discipline, motivation, and willpower. And you will fall off the wagon. Or—more specifically—into the Girl Scout cookies, which can lead into a Fuckit spiral that causes that extra bit of weight gain that statistically follows each one of these cycles. (More on the Fuckits later.)

If you want to make weight loss work for real life, if you want to create a body you are so proud of and have energy to spare, you need to make it as effortless and automated as brushing your teeth...as picking up your phone when you get a text...as covering your mouth when you cough.

You don't need more discipline, motivation, or willpower.

You need better habits.

Aristotle is often quoted as saying: "We are what we repeatedly do. Excellence, then, is not so much an act but a habit."

Notice the operative word here is "EXCELLENCE." Aristotle isn't talking about boring-ass status quo here. The word *habits* may evoke rote tasks like Mr. Rogers changing into his cardigan when he gets home, or your dad reminding you to check the oil in your car every time you fill up. But when my man Aristotle said *excellence* is a habit, he was talking about kicking some serious ass at life.

The problem is when we think of serious ass kickers, it looks like their success came in a series of "big breaks." Let's take Madonna for example. (Because who doesn't want to be Madonna?) This is what her success might look like to us:

Total unknown ➡ *Got a big break with "Holiday"* ➡ *Desperately sought Susan* ➡ *Married another celebrity, Sean Penn* ➡ *"True Blue"/"Like a Prayer" = huge hits* ➡ *Evita* ➡ *"Ray of Light"* ➡ *Highest grossing female artist of all time*

But instead, it looks like this:

Madonna worked her fucking ass off every day from 1982 until today. Period.

There's actually an article in *Psychology Today* claiming that Madonna practices her craft harder than any other celebrity, allowing her to access a state of "superfluidity." Her grueling rehearsal habit puts her actions on autopilot, which frees up her conscious brain to respond and interact with the audience. Madonna doesn't have to think about when she is supposed to kick her left leg and when she is supposed to grab her crotch. That magic just happens.

The breakout bestselling author has a daily writing habit, but we don't hear about it until it's a bestseller. Professional basketball players have shot hundreds of hoops every day for years. Michael Phelps practiced swimming every day—even on Christmas Day. You might think he pretty much has that front crawl nailed and dude could afford to take a day off. But no—the reason he excels is because of his habits.

We love the idea of a having big, dramatic weight loss and then wiping our hands on our jeans and being done with that project, but that's just not how success works. Success is the culmination of every single day when you take a tiny step toward what you want. It really doesn't happen in one dramatic episode.

Ever wonder why they've never had a *Biggest Loser* reunion show? Because it would showcase this:

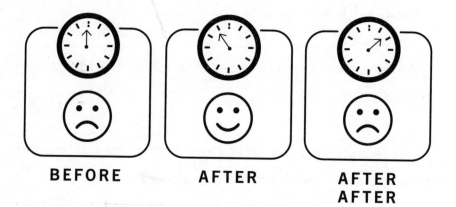

BEFORE   **AFTER**   **AFTER AFTER**

Expecting to go on a strict diet, lose a ton of weight, and then just maintain that weight loss is about as unrealistic and statistically unlikely as your retirement plan being to win the lottery, quit your job, and live off the interest. It's a great *fantasy*, but a pretty dumb *plan*.

So let's get smart. Having good habits is the health equivalent of a sensible financial plan that involves saving a little bit every day and then letting the compound interest do its freaking job. And if you are thinking that habits and compound interest don't sound very sexy and exciting, let me remind you of what happens with compound interest: it's when you get interest on the interest. So yeah—at first the growth is slow and it seems like nothing is happening, and then all of a sudden the results kick in and you are pretty much Scrooge McDuck doing laps in a swimming pool full of Benjamins.

COMPOUND INTEREST

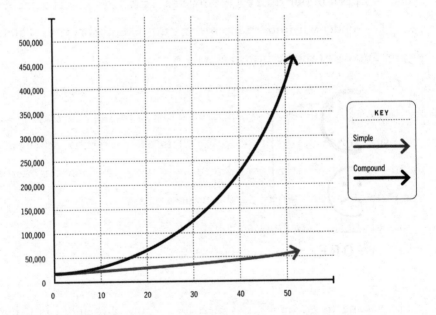

I don't know about you, but I find that chart sexy as all hell when it comes to finances. And let me tell you—it's pretty damn exciting to see the same pattern with your fitness results. You just make small changes to your everyday behaviors, and at first it seems like nothing is happening and then you hit the tipping point and you are pretty much Jennifer Lopez. (Or, you know, you feel just like her. Because remember: it's really a feeling that you are looking for.) That's the kind of compound effect that's going to happen with your fitness when you start to apply the 7 Habits of Highly Healthy Motherfuckers that I'm going to teach you.

Here's the best part: compound interest works without you having to think about it. And that's exactly why habits work so well. They don't require any extra effort or brain space. Because Madonna has the habit of practicing her craft every single day, she has all sorts of mental space left to focus on other important stuff, like pissing off religious groups and cultivating a British accent.

Once you've got your healthy habits nailed, you will have a smokin'-hot body, more energy than you ever wanted, and all the brain space you want to focus on your job, your relationship, starting your heavy metal band, whatever you want to do with your one precious life on this earth. That isn't worrying about fucking sugar.

Ready to start creating those habits?

· CHAPTER 4 ·

THE SCOOP ON
THE HABIT LOOP

THINK OF ALL THE HABITS YOU CURRENTLY HAVE AND HOW MUCH effort they take. Is it a huge pain in the ass to brush your teeth every day? Do you have to force yourself to take a shower? Do you have to motivate yourself to put on your seat belt in the car? Get inspired to check your email? Nah. I'm guessing this shit happens no matter what. You'd have to try *not* to do them.

Imagine what a pain in the ass life would be if you had to muster up the fucks to do that routine stuff every day. It would be impossible. We wouldn't get anything else done, which is why our brain is constantly scanning for routine behaviors that it can automate to save us the mental energy. It's estimated that about 40 to 45 percent of our actions are habits that we don't even think about. And just in case you don't have a PhD in fractions—that's, like, a *lot* of your life.

Bottom line: If your habits suck, you are going to feel sucky. Sucking will be your automatic default mode. If your habits rule, then you are going to feel like a queen. Being awesome will be your automatic default mode.

If you want results, stop fucking around with trendy diets and counting net carbs and instead focus on getting control of your habits, because they are running the show.

The first step in changing your habits is to understand how they work. Habits are, almost by definition, mindless, which means that most of us are completely unaware of most of our habits.

To become aware of our habits and wake the fuck up to what we are actually doing for 45 percent of our lives, it's important to understand that habits don't exist in isolation. They are prompted by a trigger and finished with a reward of some kind. Here's how it works:

First, you have the Trigger: This is what sets you off. It could be a time of day (3:00 p.m. cookie craving, anyone?), a person (we all have that friend who makes us drink a bit more wine than we should), a place (mom's house = comfort-food party time), or an emotional state (bad day at work = Bacardi night at home).

Then, you have the Behavior: This is the actual habit. Habits can be super simple (like covering your mouth when you cough or turning up the volume on the radio whenever "Hungry Like the Wolf" comes on). Or habits can be pretty complex (like driving home from work or cooking a meal that you've made a thousand times before).

Then, you have the Reward: This is the positive feeling you get from executing your habit. It could be physiological (like my beloved caffeine rush when I have my morning coffee) or psychological (like a feeling of anxiety relief when you check your email).

This Trigger-Behavior-Reward sequence is known as the habit loop. It's a loop because every time you experience the reward after performing a habit, it strengthens the relationship between the trigger and the behavior.

I'll give you a few examples that relate to weight loss and fitness:

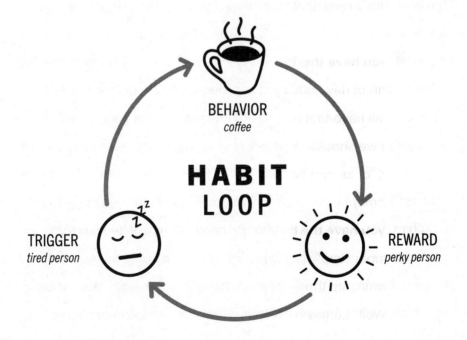

BEHAVIOR
coffee

HABIT LOOP

TRIGGER
tired person

REWARD
perky person

Trigger: You finally get the kids to sleep.

Behavior: You drink a glass of wine in front of the TV with your partner.

Reward: You experience feelings of connection, physical relaxation, and unwinding.

Trigger: It's 6:00 a.m. on a Monday, Wednesday, or Friday.

Behavior: You attend your boot-camp class.

Reward: You get exercise-induced endorphins (that's the happy drug in your brain) and feelings of self-satisfaction.

As you can see, your habits can work *for* you or *against* you.

Now that we are aware of the habit loop and how these behaviors get rooted in our brains, let's first smack down a bad habit. I'll use unconscious snacking as an example. Obviously there are worse habits out there—and as far as vices go, this is so tame that even your grandmother is bored. But if you are eating unconsciously, eventually your super hawt navel piercing is going to get buried in belly, and I'm guessing you don't want that. So let's tackle the snack monster right at the root source—your brain. In order to kill a bad habit, you have to interrupt the habit loop repeatedly until it's no longer an automated stimulus and response. We can do that by interrupting either the trigger, behavior, or reward.

I recommend working backward and first figuring out what reward you are getting from this habit. What is the need you are filling by wandering to the fridge? Are you looking for an energetic boost? Are you just bored and looking to do something with your hands? Are you avoiding doing something else that is uncomfortable? Are you feeling down on yourself and need to feel loved and treated? Once you've figured out the need you are trying to fill from this habit, you can replace the behavior with something that will do the trick without sabotaging your health goals. If you are looking for an energy boost, you can replace the cookie habit with a green tea or twenty jumping jacks and get the same reward. If you need to keep your hands busy, I have many clients who have knitted their way into smaller jeans because it kept their hands out of the chip bag in the evenings. (Bonus: Scarves for everyone!)

If you are looking to feel loved and treated, this is where you have to dig a little deeper to find something that isn't a cookie to genuinely make you feel the same way. What will scratch that emotional itch for a little indulgence?

This is inner work that no one else can do but you—but here are a few ideas: you could maybe substitute a quick text exchange with a friend, or ask your boo for a hug, take a break from work and treat yourself to a musical interlude with your favorite song, surf the net for pics of your next vacation, take a deep breath and think of three things you are grateful for. Even substituting an orange for the cookie is a step in the right direction if it genuinely makes you feel treated. (Even though the habit of eating when you want to feel loved will still be in place, every small win counts, as we will discuss further in chapter 9: "If You Can't Do Something Right, Do It Totally Half-Ass.")

But really the most effective way to pulverize a bad habit is to eliminate the trigger. Unfortunately, that is easier said than done, as often your trigger is going to be emotional—usually boredom or stress. So here's where you are going to have to do some soul searching again: What can you do to make your life more interesting or less stressful? Seriously. I had clients who would say things like "I don't know what's wrong with me—I'm just so run off my feet and I can't stop snacking!" And I'm thinking, *This isn't a snacking problem; this is a LIFE problem. You don't need weight-loss advice; you need to figure out how to make your life easier.*

I know you just want me to tell you to replace your cookie with celery sticks or whatever, but if celery sticks don't alleviate your stress, it's not going to give you the reward you need and your willpower won't last. If you want to get lean and Healthy as Fuck, you are going to have to come to grips with the fact that you need to do the *real* work of figuring out what triggers you and what rewards you need—rather than the *easy* work of just following a meal plan and chomping on some celery because some trainer told you to.

> **Do the real work of figuring out what triggers you and what rewards you need—rather than the easy work of just following a meal plan.**

On the other hand, if the trigger is environmental, this is fairly easy to circumvent. Don't go to that coffee shop with the excellent muffins. Don't hang out with that person who is always like "It's five o'clock somewhere!" as they fish around for the big wineglasses.

If you always snack on the couch and watch TV—instead, brush your teeth, go to bed, and watch your show there (yeah yeah, it's not great for sleep, but one thing at a time). People are often most successful at changing their habits when they move to a new environment. So if you have any shifts in your job or housing coming up, this is a great time to be intentional about building your new habits. If not, I tell you how to shake up your environment and set yourself up for success in chapter 6: "The Life-Changing, Magical Art of Getting Your Shit Together."

Either way, now is the time to consciously create your new healthy habits that are going to totally transform your bod and your life. Here's how:

1. **Choose the habit you want to cultivate.**

I humbly suggest you consider one of the 7 Habits of Highly Healthy Motherfuckers that we'll get to in the next chapter.

2. **Then, choose your trigger.**

What's going to set off your awesome new habit? The best idea is to hang your new habit on an existing circumstance that is nonnegotiable. Be sure to make your trigger:

Specific: "Right after I shower" is better than "every morning."
Consistent: "When I get to work" is not a good trigger if you are

a freelancer with irregular work hours and locations. "As soon as I wake up" would be a better one because it happens every day no matter what.

Logical: "When my kids go to bed" is not a logical time to work out if you get tired in the evenings. "After I've answered all my emails" is not a logical time to meditate since Inbox Zero is a magical, mythical fairy tale. Instead, try "Right after I've had my coffee" for your workout. "Right after I get dressed" might be a more realistic time to meditate.

Here are some examples of triggers that tend to work well as anchors because they are the types of actions we tend to do consistently and mark a specific moment in each day:

As soon as I wake up

After my shower

While I make coffee

When I walk my dog

On my drive to work

After lunch

After I pick up my kids

When I change into my pajamas

When I get in bed

3. **Figure out the reward.**

Most of the 7 Habits of Highly Healthy Motherfuckers that I'm about to teach you will have their own intrinsic reward. Eventually. Like, you know, the sense of oneness with the Universe when you meditate for twenty years. But, like compound interest, that shit might not kick in right away, so you should totally bribe yourself into good behavior until it does.

I definitely needed a bribe when I first started exercising. I don't know about you, but when these perky girls would talk about the "runner's high" I thought they were actually high, because my first heaving attempts at running felt like twenty minutes of psychological misery and physical hell, and I spent the whole time desperately trying to think of a reason why it would be okay if I stopped.

Until I found a reward that worked for me.

I promised myself that I could watch WHATEVER HORRIBLE MIND-ROTTING CRAP I wanted as long as I did it while power walking/ jogging on a treadmill. I felt so naughty as I caught every paternity test on Maury Povich and furtively turned up the volume on *Grease 2*.

Now I exercise because it makes me feel amazing immediately afterward, but that wasn't always the case. It used to totally suck. But it definitely sucked less when Maury got those lie-detector test results back, youknowwhatI'msayin'?

Stop trying to convince yourself that you'll execute your new habit just because you SHOULD. If that was the case, you'd already have all this shit on lockdown and Beyoncé would be pinning pictures of YOUR legs for inspiration.

There are tons of studies that show that rewards are highly effective to reinforce positive behaviors. Without the reward, the loop is incomplete and the behavior will always be an effort instead of automatic. This is the way our brains work, so just roll with it and reward yourself, mmmkay?

Now, this is where you get to do some soul searching (yes, more soul searching—deal with it) to figure out both (1) what makes you feel rewarded and (2) what is also a health-positive behavior (or at least health-neutral). If your new habit is to go for a thirty-minute walk after dinner, but your reward is to then drink Bud until you pass out, I don't know if you are going to end up ahead in the health and wellness game. The best reward is something:

Immediate. It has to be something you can consistently deliver right after or during your habit. If you get up at 6:00 a.m. to exercise and then promise yourself an afternoon nap as a reward, your brain won't make the association between the two actions—and it won't form an automatic habit loop.

Actually feels like a reward. For example, if you try to "reward" yourself with half an apple after choking down an undressed kale salad, your brain will call bullshit if it doesn't feel like enough of a treat to reinforce the habit. One reward that works for me is saving my delicious breakfast smoothie until after my workout.

Only you know what will make you feel rewarded. But here are some ideas that have worked for others:

- Download new music.
- Use an app that tracks your progress so you can see a satisfying streak that you won't want to break.
- Post your triumph and awesomeness on social media and bask in the admiration of your peers.
- Make the habit more fun and social by involving friends.
- Allow yourself ten minutes in the sauna in your gym or a quiet sit on a park bench after your run.
- Enjoy some guilt-free online window shopping/Pinterest browsing.
- Take some alone time with a great book.
- Connect with a long-distance friend.
- Invest in a Fitbit or some other cool gear.
- Listen to your favorite podcast while you go for a walk.

Okay. So now you know how to consciously create a new habit, but not all habits are created equal. What you want to get to work on are the 7 Habits of Highly Healthy Motherfuckers.

· CHAPTER 5 ·

THE 7 HABITS OF HIGHLY HEALTHY MOTHERFUCKERS

I HAD A FRIEND WHO WORKED FOR THE FAST-FOOD CHAIN Wendy's. She once told me a story about the person who came in and ordered a Baconator combo with chili cheese nachos, a vanilla Frosty... and a *Diet* Coke. We would giggle at the preposterousness of the last-ditch attempt at caloric restraint. Ridiculous, right?

But I wonder if this sounds more familiar: the person who goes to the latest trendy restaurant and is careful to send the bread basket away, order the grass-fed organic beef, and trade the potato for a salad with the dressing on the side...and then orders three artisanal cocktails—double shots in each with simple syrup and a maraschino cherry.

Don't get me wrong—this makes a LOT of sense in a foodie, deliciousness kind of way. But not really from a health perspective.

It would have been way healthier for that person to have the damn potato and skip the third cocktail.

People are more conscious and health focused than ever before. But they are focusing on the wrong things. And usually that's because of the wellness news cycle churning out more breaking stories about health and fitness, keeping us distracted by the latest super-foods and bro-science instead of just living our lives and focusing on the basics.

Because the things you actually need to focus on are old news. Boring. Imagine trying to sell magazines with a big headline saying *Vegetables! Still good for you after all these years!*

Instead, it's much more profitable to headline some breaking news about *Ice cream is low on the glycemic index!* (This is true, by the way—the protein and fat slow down the absorption of sugar.)

But investing your health efforts in the relatively low glycemic index of ice cream would be an example of focusing on the wrong thing.

Sure, there are a gazillion healthy habits that are worth cultivating. Taking a multivitamin probably isn't a bad idea. Good posture never hurt anyone. Want to chew your food ninety-nine times before you swallow? Knock yourself out.

But keep in mind that we have a limited amount of fucks to give about this—so I say we distribute those fucks in the smartest way possible, and that is keystone habits.

In architecture, a keystone is defined as "a central stone at the summit of an arch, locking the whole together."

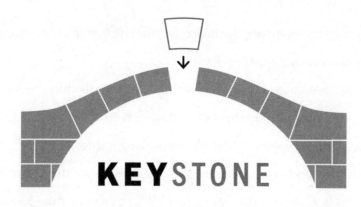

KEYSTONE

In behavior, a keystone habit is one that sets off a snowball effect of other positive behaviors.

For example: I exercise first thing in the morning. I know that makes me a little bit hateable, and maybe you are one of the many who would rather gouge out their eyes with a fork than exercise first thing in the morning. But check out the ripple effect. When I exercise first thing in the morning:

- I don't really *want* to have three coffees and a pastry for breakfast; I want to eat something nourishing.
- I am awake and energetic and motivated to pack a healthy lunch.
- I have already finished my workout, so I have more time to spend with my kids in the evening.
- I am less likely to have drinks in the evening and more likely to go to bed on time because I've got to get up early to work out.

So, it's not that I'm fit because my workout burns all these calories. I'm fit because the workout sets off a chain reaction of healthy behaviors that add up to me being the insanely hot MILF you see on the inside cover of this book.

In focusing on keystone habits, I'm applying the 80/20 rule—also known as the Pareto Principle. The Pareto Principle states that we get 80 percent of our results from 20 percent of our effort. For example, in business, 80 percent of sales will usually come from 20 percent of the clients. In baseball, it was observed that 80 percent of the wins came from the top 20 percent of the players.

In health and fitness, 80 percent of your results are going to come from 20 percent of your efforts. The trick is to figure out what is the 20 percent effort that is actually delivering results, and then just do more of that.

I call them the **7 Keystone Habits of Highly Healthy Motherfuckers**.

HABIT #1: FILL HALF OF EVERY PLATE WITH VEGETABLES

Want a new diet that actually works?

Fill half of every plate with vegetables. That's it. That is your new nutrition plan. You can stop stressing about carbs and fat and protein and gluten and turmeric and whatever. Instead, aim for about seven servings of vegetables a day and watch your belly shrink, your moods regulate, and your health improve. Not only will you get hella hot and feel like a sexy MOFO, you'll add years onto your life just by filling half of every plate with vegetables.

I know it sounds too simple, but it's actually a huge shift from the way most people eat, even if they think they already eat very healthy.

Research shows that only 9 percent of Americans are eating the amount of vegetables recommended by the World Health Organization (WHO).

It's not at all uncommon for me to have a client who claims to have a great diet, and when I look at their food journal it looks like this:

Breakfast: Whole grain granola and plain Greek yogurt with
   a banana

Lunch: Chicken and avocado on a gluten-free wrap

Snack: "Clean" protein bar

Dinner: Salmon with quinoa pilaf and side of asparagus

Now, I don't want to shit all over this menu, because it's not like this person is snorting lines of trans fats and pouring vodka over their Cheerios. They are clearly making an effort—and I'm assuming if you are reading a book like this, then *you* are clearly making an effort. I'm just saying that if you want to focus on the 20 percent effort that delivers 80 percent results, then you should shift that effort to focus on VEGETABLES.

The menu outlined above (which contains only one serving of vegetables…two, if there were a tomato thrown into that wrap) is what I often see from my clients who have been trying to offload the last few pounds for the better half of their lives. When they switch to a more vegetable-centered approach, then the weight falls off and they feel so much better.

Here's an example of the focus shift I'm suggesting.

When you stand in front of the fridge to plan a meal, you probably start with the protein, right? "Okay, so we'll have some chicken...and then on the side we'll have some rice...and I should probably use up that cauliflower."

Or maybe you are a plant-based eater and you start with the starch: "We'll have buckwheat soba noodles, and then on top we'll throw some peppers and onions."

Here's what I want. When you open your fridge, you should hear the song "Welcome to the Jungle" in your head because there are so many freaking plants in there. Then, when you are mentally constructing your meal, the first thought that goes through your head should be something like *Now, which vegetables will I fill half my plate with?*

To get you all fired up about getting your veggies in, consider this:

- Vegetables are the one thing that pretty much every diet has ever agreed upon.

  Unless the diet is just totally stupid (like the Cotton-Ball Diet, where you soak cotton balls in liquid and eat them to make yourself full—this seriously happened; don't freaking try it, obvi), every diet trend has basically been a variation of (1) eat more vegetables, but also (2) DO THIS BRAND-NEW THING. Diet books are sold on the supposed revolutionary new findings about macronutrient distribution or superfoods, but open any of them and the real "secret" is replacing a lot of processed crap with a *lot* of green.

- Vegetables are low in calories. If you are eating mostly vegetables, you basically can't overeat. Try it. I freaking *dare* you to try to have a broccoli binge. It's nature's "points system," where the points come from your *own body* saying "Holy fuck, dude. That's too much broccoli. Can we just chill?"

Vegetables are little phytochemical bombs of awesomeness. Phytochemicals are what gives the food it's color (that's why you are always being told to eat a rainbow), and they are powerful antioxidant agents. Research suggests that phytochemicals help prevent cardiovascular disease, cancer, type 2 diabetes, and age-related mental decline. Seriously—if you could get a patent on a pill that was as powerful as just eating plants, you'd be hella rich.

- Vegetables are high in dietary fiber. You care because dietary fiber keeps you feeling full on fewer calories and without eating a bunch of bullshit. Dietary fiber also lowers your cholesterol, stabilizes your blood sugar, and helps you poo (which is basically instant weight loss, so what's not to love?).

Vegetables are packed with vitamins and minerals. Vitamins and minerals are organic compounds that your body needs to function normally, and you need to get them from food. If you aren't getting the vitamins and minerals you need, then not only do you risk chronic health conditions, you will look and feel like total shit.

Oh? But you don't *like* vegetables? Do you like energy, a hot bod, and living a long time? Then I suggest you get into vegetables. That's what I advised this guy who hired me to help him drop some weight and maximize his sports performance, but warned me, "Just to let you know, I don't like vegetables, so you've got your work cut out for you, Duncan."

To which I replied, "Actually, you've got *your* work cut out for you. Because you are about to completely change your life by eating a lot of vegetables."

My point here is that you are an adult, and you are responsible for your own choices. Eat what you want, but if you are reading this to get healthy and hot, you are going to be eating a shit ton of vegetables—and they don't have to taste like mushy, chlorophyll-plant-matter punishment. Vegetables can be as delicious as Brad Pitt's debut in *Thelma and Louise*. If you don't believe me, go to my site (www.fitfeelsgood.com/book) and grab some of my free recipes, and you'll see why that dude was eating his words (and his kale) in twenty-eight days and thanking me.

But what about protein?

A recent study shows that 60 percent of Americans are now actively trying to increase their protein consumption. This is total bonkerstown. Repeat after me: "I really don't need more protein." In Canada and the United States, the average person is consuming nearly twice as much protein as recommended. Another way to say that is that the average person is consuming WAY too many calories in excess protein.

And yes, you can gain weight from protein. Because protein has been marketed as a health food, people have this idea that it's "free"—that they can consume as much of it as they want without gaining weight.

This is also a tenet of the keto/paleo movement and part of what makes it so popular. It's absolutely insane. Protein has four calories per gram. Carbohydrates also have four calories per gram. If you are overconsuming protein (and, according to the WHO, you probably are—by a *lot*), then that is a just a lot of calories you don't need. A generation of people have been sold on the idea that carbs make you fat, and protein makes you lean. This is a lie. Excess calories make you fat. A caloric deficit makes you lean. A gram of protein and a gram of carbohydrate have the same number of calories. Overeating any kind of food will make you gain weight. More on that later.

Nonetheless, the marketing of more protein = healthier is probably one of the most successful food fads of our time. A 2014 market research report showed that consumers will spend more money on their food if the word *protein* is emphasized. A perfect example of the health-washing of protein is the Cantina Power Menu at Taco Bell, which boasts double the meat for "twenty grams of protein!" The company president is quoted as saying, "People are looking for food that gives them energy."

This shows that people are completely confused about what protein actually does. Protein doesn't give you energy. Carbohydrates give you energy. Protein's job is to build and repair muscles and tissues. When you work out, you put stress on your muscles and create little microtears. Protein's job is to help your body to repair that muscle and make it bigger and stronger—WHEN YOU WORK OUT. You can't just sit in your car scarfing protein bars and think that you are building muscle. What you are doing is consuming excess calories and gaining weight. Stop it. Swap your protein bar for carrot and celery sticks, and if you want to build muscle, then, um, use your muscles (more on that coming up).

Don't get me wrong—I'm not starting a new "evil macronutrient" campaign here by saying that we should avoid all protein (although damn, dude—if I were successful with starting a new anti-protein diet trend, I could make a trillion dollars with new food products with big, healthy-looking seals promising that this Twinkie is "Protein-Free!"). I'm just pointing out that most people are *way* overconsuming protein and way underconsuming vegetables. Reversing that trend and consuming everything in appropriate portions (specifics comin' up) will make you a hell of a lot leaner and healthier.

Here's a sample day's menu in which half of every meal is vegetables. This meets the seven servings of vegetables and three servings of fruit recommended by a recent meta-analysis done by Imperial College London.

Breakfast: Carrot-cake smoothie: banana, some oats, a big-ass handful of spinach, a carrot or two, a couple of walnuts, some dates to sweeten it, and a splash of almond milk to lube it all up. Maybe chuck in some cinnamon and vanilla if they happen to be within reach.

Lunch: Lentil vegetable soup, and apple for dessert

Snack: Celery with almond butter

Dinner: Zucchini, cherry tomatoes, and tofu tossed in sundried-tomato pesto with long-grain brown rice and a bowl of berries for dessert

By the way, this menu provides 62 grams of plant-based protein—more than enough for an active, medium-sized woman in her forties. According to the World Health Organization, 0.83 grams of protein per kilo of body weight is sufficient for 97.5 percent of the population. And it's totally possible (in fact—better) to meet all your protein needs by eating plants. But seriously, before you bust out your calculator and start tracking your food to figure out your grams, let me just tell you: Protein is almost definitely not a problem for you. Even if you go to the gym. Even if you are vegan. Fussing about calculating your protein grams would be an example of busywork, the kind of easy effort that wastes time and distracts people from actually making real change in their bodies. It's really way less complicated than the fitness marketing cycle would have you think.

If you do love numbers and research, ditch the protein-obsessed bro-science and look at the largest and most comprehensive study on human nutrition ever done: the China Study.

Called the "Grand Prix of epidemiology" by the *New York Times*, the China Study was a partnership between Cornell University, Oxford University, and the Chinese Academy of Preventive Medicine. It collated massive amounts of data collected over a span of twenty years. Here's what they figured out: "People who ate the most plant-based foods were the healthiest."

They recommend going straight up vegan (which is what I did as soon as I learned this information), but even if that's not your jam, T. Colin Campbell, called the Einstein of Nutrition, recommends putting as many plants on your plate as possible to avoid disease and get to a healthy body weight.

Which is why I say you start with filling half of every plate with veggies as your new #1 Keystone Habit. If you make that one change, you can ditch all the rest of your complicated food rules and get on with your life.

Your long (lean) and healthy life.

Now, even if you aren't salivating at the thought of more cauliflower, I know this next keystone habit will get you excited...

HABIT #2: GO THE FUCK TO SLEEP

It's not exactly breaking news that you are totally screwed without a good sleep—and the world is finally catching on. Sheryl Sandberg of *Lean In* fame rocked the business world by recommending that executives prioritize sleep over working more. The Dalai Lama claims that sleep is the best meditation there is. Actor Mindy Kaling is quoted as saying, "There is no sunrise so beautiful that it is worth waking me up to see it." When I mention to my clients that we are going to be focusing on sleep as much as burpees, they almost weep with relief. And here's why—since 1960, chronic sleep deprivation has increased dramatically in North America. If you are regularly getting less than seven hours of sleep a night, you are in that bleary-eyed club. And don't even go telling me that you are perfectly fine on five hours. Science says you are kidding yourself—just like the tipsy guy who thinks he is totally fine to drive.

Everyone needs at least seven hours of sleep a night in order to function optimally. You also need those forty winks if you are going to lose your belly. Here are four reasons why.

Lack of sleep produces cortisol.

When you are sleep deprived, your body assumes that you aren't sleeping because you must be in some kind of crisis. And when in crisis, the body creates a hormone called cortisol to help you get through it. It's the fight-or-flight hormone that helped keep our ancestors alive during times of stress—when stress meant we had to flee from a saber-toothed tiger or survive a famine or something. In those cases, it was really helpful that cortisol sent the body into lockdown mode, slowing down the metabolism and storing fat around the middle in order to help us survive the plague or Mongolian raiders or whatever.

In modern times that translates to you lying awake in bed, stressing about whether you are going to make it to Costco tomorrow before it gets too busy, and dumbass cortisol thinking, *She's probably stressed that the continents have shifted and there aren't enough mammoths to go around. I should probably make her fatter!* Thanks, cortisol, you dick.

A lack of sleep basically makes you drunk.

Guess what? If you've been awake for eighteen hours, you have the motor and cognitive impairment of someone who has a blood alcohol concentration of 0.08 percent, which is legally drunk (and leaves you at equal risk for a crash, btw).

And when you are drunk, do you eat lots of vegetables and make fantastic decisions for your health? No, you do not. You eat chili cheese fries and watch Netflix HARD.

Sleep is when you reap the benefits of your workout.

When you exercise, you put stress on your body. But it's the good kind of stress, the what-doesn't-kill-me-makes-me-stronger stress. The stress part happens in the gym when you are on your sixty-third squat and your quads are begging for mercy. But the getting stronger part happens later that night when you're sleeping. Deep sleep releases growth hormone, which not only builds and repairs muscles and tissue, but prevents premature aging. Without the sleep, you've just got...stress. And (as I will repeat ad infinitum) stress will make you retain fat and be generally miserable.

Lack of sleep gives you the crazy munchies.

When you sleep, the body balances two hunger-controlling hormones, ghrelin (makes you hungry) and leptin (makes you feel satisfied). If you get less than six hours of sleep, your ghrelin levels rise, and your leptin is repressed, meaning you are going to want that second piece of cake. And maybe the third. And then you might have trouble metabolizing that cake due to a sleep-deprived overproduction of insulin, which can lead to—you guessed it—body fat storage. (Also increased risk of diabetes, but who's counting?)

Good sleep boosts your immune system and keeps you ready to move.

A lack of sleep can make you prone to getting colds and the flu, which is exactly the kind of thing that's going to prevent you from being consistent with your training program. When you are well-rested and healthy, you are good to go for a wicked workout, which is in turn going to help you sleep better later on, inducing a positive cycle.

When you're sleeping, you aren't snacking.

Best way to shut your pie hole? Shut your eyes. When people ask me about the best snacks to have at night, I'll usually tell them (with love): "If you are craving snacks at night, that's probably because you are *tired* and your body is screaming for energy. Skip *The Late Show* and go the fuck to sleep."

But sometimes going the fuck to sleep is easier said than done. If you are like a lot of my clients, you are a huge fan of sleep. If sleep were a teen heartthrob, you'd have its picture hanging in your locker with puffy-heart stickers. The only problem is that sleep, like a teen heartthrob, can sometimes be a bit elusive. Either you can't get yourself to wind down at the end of the day, or you wake up at 3:00 a.m. with a spinning mind. If you want *you + sleep = true love 4eva*, here's what you need to do:

1. Stay regular.

    Go to sleep and get up at the same time every day. Even on weekends. Yup, you heard me. Don't try to "catch up" on sleep by sleeping in on weekends—you are just screwing yourself

over to ever feel rested because your body won't be able to find
its rhythm. Establish a routine to wind yourself down and stick
to it so the body starts to recognize when it's night-night time.

2. Keep your workouts and your caffeine early.

    We all know that a great workout will give you an energy
    and endorphin boost. This is awesome at 9:00 a.m., but not
    so welcome at 9:00 p.m. Ideally, your workout will end at
    least two hours before it's time to start your bedtime routine.
    However, the most recent studies show that exercise at any time
    of day will promote a better sleep than not exercising at all, so
    I'm afraid you don't get to ditch your evening workout in the
    name of better z's. You might want to skip that afternoon coffee
    though. Try to limit caffeine and have the last cup of coffee
    before 2:00 p.m. Don't fall for that afternoon treat business
    from Starbucks. That's just The Man fucking with you.

3. If you can't sleep, get up.

    Give yourself twenty minutes of restlessness and contem-
    plating climate change and wondering what your high-school
    crush is doing and then get up, change the scenery, and do
    something quiet like read a book or have a magnesium-rich
    snack like a banana. (That's not random; magnesium helps you
    sleep. Spinach is also full of magnesium, but no one is getting
    out of bed for spinach, amiright?)

4. Get outside.

    I'm a huge believer in getting outside as often as possible, which is why I bully all my clients to get thirty minutes of outdoors time every day. Studies show that exposure to sunlight can help regulate circadian rhythms—the internal body clock that decides when it's time to sleep and when it's time to party. If your workplace is a cubical cave of fluorescent light, you need to be especially careful to get outdoors during your breaks. (Tip: follow the smokers. They are so outdoorsy!)

5. Step away from your phone an hour before lights out.

    The clicky-clicky temptations of your screens are not telling your body it's time to wind down. They are telling you that everyone has a nicer house than you and you should probably buy new shoes immediately. Get old school with a book or a magazine... or another pleasant bedroom activity of your choosing (*wink*).

6. Lay off the booze.

    Stop kidding yourself that your nightly glass (*cough* half bottle *cough*) of wine is helping you sleep at night. Oh sure, it will get you to bed—but after you pass out, the quality of your sleep will be shitty. You won't get the REM sleep (deep sleep) you need for maximum mental and physical regeneration, and you'll probably wake up in the middle of the night and have trouble dozing off again.

In fact, laying off the booze is so important that it's a keystone habit all on its own. So put that corkscrew away, turn on the kettle, and settle in for Habit #3...

HABIT #3: BACK AWAY FROM THE BOOZE

I wish I didn't have to type that, but I really do. I get that there's nothing better than a glass of wine after a hard day. It feels like a reward for doing LIFE. Which is why when I was pregnant and hung out with other pregnant ladies, one of the hot topics was alcohol.

> "Is it really so bad to have a little sip?"
>
> "How awful is it that I got drunk on New Year's Eve before I found out that I was pregnant?"
>
> "This baby is about to fall out of me. Surely it can't do any harm to have a drink *now*?"

I asked my midwife about it and she responded with "No amount of alcohol has been proven safe for the baby." (*sad trombone*)

But here's the real kick in the pants: That is still the case long after you are born. No amount of alcohol has been proven to be safe. For any of us. Now, before you decide that this book might actually be better used as a nice coaster, let me tell you this: I'm not going to tell you that you have to abstain from all alcohol. Instead, I am going to tell you that there's a good chance you are drinking too much. And there's a really good chance that it's affecting your fitness results.

When I was in my twenties, my doctor asked me how many alcoholic drinks I had in a week. "Seven," I answered confidently, because I had heard that seven was the recommended limit for women. What I didn't tell her—and she didn't ask—was that all seven were happening on Friday night (in amazing gold lamé American Apparel leggings, thank you very much). Consuming that much alcohol in a single night is actually considered binge drinking if you want to get all pedantic about it, and we all know that's not particularly good for you blah blah blah.

Now I'm all grown up. I've retired those leggings, and those Friday nights are ancient history (see reference above re: pregnancy). So you can imagine my indignation when I learned that my new, terribly sophisticated adult drinking habits actually qualified me to be a "heavy drinker."

WHAT.

If you had asked me, I would have said my drinking habits were normal—and they probably are. Tell me if you can relate to this:

Sometimes a girl likes to unwind with a small glass of wine at least three nights a week. Totally normal, right? So according to the United States Dietary Guidelines Advisory Committee, that qualifies as a "moderate drinker."

Fine. I'm comfortable with that.

But let's get realistic and say you actually have a glass of wine pretty much every night. Sometimes maybe that glass isn't so small, but more like a bowl with a stem on it. And at some point during the weekend you will definitely enjoy a cocktail or two. Now, those United States Dietary Guideline killjoys are graduating you to the category of "heavy drinker," according to the recommended guidelines for women. Heavy drinker? Come ON! That seems a little alarmist, right? It's not like I'm doing tequila shots in line at the bank and showing up for school pickup wearing one of those beer-funnel hats! The kind of drinking I do is just called grown-up LIFE! Who's with me, ladies?!

A *lot* of ladies are with me. Alcohol used to be marketed with sex, romance, adventure, sophistication. But a few years ago the conversation shifted, and suddenly "Mommy Juice" is just something you need to get through the freaking week. It's just *fun* to give your friend a wine-dispensing purse. Adding a greeting card is easy because about a third of the cards aimed at women will include sassy jokes like "Who is this 'Moderation' we're supposed to be drinking with?" or "A day without wine is like...just kidding, I have no idea!"

Okay, those are kind of funny. But it's not funny how much we are all drinking and how it's affecting our health—and waistlines. In her book, *Drink*, Ann Dowsett Johnston talks about how alcohol use in women in the developed world has skyrocketed over the past decade. And here's the thing—just because it's normal doesn't mean it's good. It's also normal to be feeling the consequences of drinking too much. By the time most of my clients get to me, they are starting to feel that nightly glass of wine affecting their energy and their mood. And they are certainly feeling it when they try to zip up their pants.

I'm sure I'm not going to shock you by saying that alcohol is a horrible idea if you are trying to lose weight. I mean, you know it's high in calories with zero nutrition. It stimulates appetite. It is high in sugar, which triggers an insulin response, which can lead to fat storage, particularly around the middle. It decreases the quality of your sleep, which (as you've seen) also makes you gain weight. And it makes you less inhibited around food and very unlikely to work out the next day. I hate to say it, but that nightly glass of wine really leads to a total shit storm for belly fat. Oh—and cancer and all that as well.

A recent paper published in New Zealand showed that a third of alcohol-related cancer deaths among women were associated with less than two standard drinks per day. But what about all those delightful viral articles in your Facebook feed that talk about the health benefits of red wine and that if you lived in Tuscany and started drinking wine with lunch when you were eight years old you would live to be one hundred?

Here's what those studies are talking about: There is an interesting relationship between alcohol and health risk that results in a J-shaped curve, like the one pictured on the next page. If you look closely, you'll see that heavy drinkers have a high risk of mortality—obvi. But you'll also see that absolute abstainers also have an uptick in their relative risk of mortality, while moderate drinkers have the lowest risk of early mortality.

BUT. That doesn't prove moderate drinking is the cause of lower mortality. Just because there's a correlation between moderate drinking and longevity, it doesn't mean there is a causal relationship. Maybe there are other factors at play. Maybe moderate drinkers are also happier, more social, or less stressed out. Maybe absolute abstainers are abstaining because they are already sick or have previous addiction issues and that's why they don't touch the stuff.

J CURVE

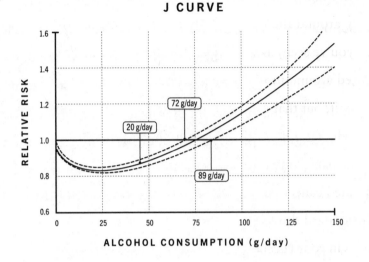

Just because one variable (moderate drinking) seems to be related to another (maximum life span) doesn't mean it's directly affecting the other variable. Here's another great example of correlation vs. causation:

Number of People Who Drowned by Falling into a Swimming Pool

correlates with

Number of Films Nicolas Cage Appeared In

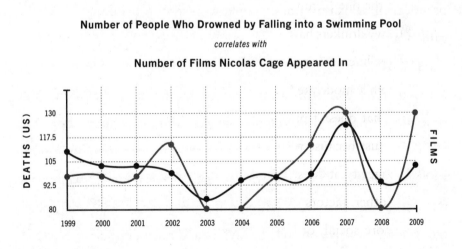

...just sayin'.

Like I said, all that stuff about antioxidants in red wine is (sadly) not the reality. Remember, there was a time when doctors were recommending brands of cigarettes ("The touch of menthol added to Kool cigarettes soothes the throat!"). In my opinion, the dubious claims of fringe health benefits are historically the last gasp of an industry that is getting busted for harming us. According to the Center for Disease Control: "The risk of death from cancer appears to go up with any level of alcohol consumption. The current and emerging science does not support the purported benefits of moderate drinking."

Which is why seven drinks a week for women is the LIMIT. Not recommended dosage. You'll never hear a doctor recommend you START drinking if you don't already. Having guidelines of how much of a toxic substance is acceptable is called *risk management*. Doctors came up with these limits because in most cases it's not practical or realistic to ask people to just stop drinking. I feel the same way.

This is where I get to the part where I tell you that you don't necessarily have to stop drinking. Yes, the latest studies show that absolute abstinence is probably the best thing for your body, but we are more than just bodies. That's why my favorite definition of wellness is from my personal trainer certification course: "Wellness is the search for enhanced quality of life, personal growth, and potential through positive lifestyle behaviors and attitudes."

I love this definition because:

- It talks about quality of life being the ultimate goal rather than a body-fat percentage or bio age or other statistic.
- It defines wellness as a "search for" and "growth" rather than an end point.
- It takes into account your attitude, which is everything.

So, in my opinion, if occasional alcohol is the social lubricant you need to get up and dance at the wedding, or an integral part of a cherished cultural ritual that's been around for generations, or the perfect enhancer to a holiday meal, I don't think it's necessarily "better" to abstain.

However, if you want to be Healthy as Fuck, you are going to have to face up to how much you are drinking—and *why* you are drinking. Here's what I want you to do:

Take an honest, nonjudgy tally of how much you are currently drinking per week.

Have a think: What alcohol do you consume habitually that you could survive without? Is it:

The third drink at the bar on Friday?

The glass of wine while you prep dinner every night?

The B52 shot you licked off that guy's belly at your friend's bachelorette party?

Which are the drinks that contribute to your quality of life? And which are the ones that are moving you further away?

Now that you've given some thought to the amount of alcohol that serves you best (remember—*you* always get to choose!), here are some ideas on how to reduce your intake without going nuts.

Destroy the habit loop by interrupting the trigger.

Remember that the structure of a habit is trigger, behavior, reward. Which booze triggers can you consciously avoid or interrupt? For example, if you tend to drink a glass of wine while you watch TV at night, interrupt the trigger by brushing your teeth and taking a book to bed. If you tend to meet your girlfriends for dinner and drinks, switch it to brunch and a walk.

Exchange the habit loop for a better one by replacing the behavior.

As we've already discussed, it's easy enough to avoid triggers if they are environmental, but emotional triggers are trickier. Stress is probably the biggest trigger for wanting a drink, and not totally avoidable. So what you need to do is replace the behavior you carry out in response to the trigger and try to get a similar reward.

You might think that nothing is going to chill you out as effectively as a nice glass of wine, but as Annie Grace points out in her brilliant book, *This Naked Mind*, we have the illusion that alcohol reduces stress, when it actually just numbs the feeling temporarily. As soon as the effects of the drink wear off, we're left contending with alcohol withdrawal as well as the original reason we are stressed out, which leads to wanting another drink. And then you wake up the next morning after a shitty sleep with a hangover and are much less able to cope with whatever is stressing you out. In the long run, alcohol will always make stress worse.

On top of that, when you reach for the bottle every time you are stressed, you rob yourself of the opportunity to figure out how to self-soothe. Only you can figure out what will genuinely make you feel better after a rough day. The bubble bath cliché? Masturbating? Watching *Labyrinth* with David Bowie? Watching *Labyrinth* with David Bowie while masturbating in the bath? Now *that* is a Tuesday night.

Experiment with clear parameters around booze.

Annie Grace has a great Thirty-Day Alcohol Experiment, in which you abstain from all alcohol for thirty days to see how you feel. She also gives great information and context to help you reframe your beliefs about alcohol. If working on your relationship to booze is a goal for you and you are looking for some structure around a Dry January, this is a highly recommended (and totally free) program.

As I mentioned, I don't insist on absolute abstinence for my clients but suggest the following parameters:

- No alcohol at all during the week.
- Go ahead and drink once a weekend during your "treat meal." Limit to two drinks.

- Only drink "happy" alcohol. Use it as an enhancement to celebrate in good company. Never as a Band-Aid solution for a bad mood. If you hear yourself thinking *I need a drink* in a grumpy way, then you know it isn't happy booze, and it's a great moment of self-awareness to see if you can experiment with an alternate coping mechanism. (And truth? Sometimes you'll experiment with an alternate like the whole Davie Bowie bath situation and you'll still want the glass of wine. Either way, you are awesome for conducting the experiment and being awake and aware of how you are feeling—rather than just reflexively grabbing the wine. That, my friend, is doing the real work of getting Healthy as Fuck.)

Using those guidelines, people all over the world have successfully shifted from a daily glass of wine to cope to a weekly glass of wine to *celebrate*. In doing so, they have saved themselves countless calories, deepened their sleep, increased their energy, taken a major step toward getting rid of a stubborn belly, and reduced their risk of cancer. Seriously. When you back away from the booze, you are taking a giant step toward your new life as a Healthy Motherfucker.

HABIT #4: CHILL YOUR ASS OUT (AND MEDITATE)

I know you might not believe me, but it's possible that all you need to do in order to achieve your fitness goals is…less.

Less striving. Less effort. But most of all, less stress.

I learned this the hard way during my early years as a fitness instructor. As I've mentioned, I was a bit of a late bloomer in the whole fitness department, so I had the fervor of the recently converted. I was teaching several high-intensity classes a day, training for a half marathon, as well as working on my yoga teaching certification. I was still a little chubby, so I had impostor syndrome in my new career. But I figured if I just worked a little harder, then I would get the body I thought a real fitness professional should have. And then my yoga instructor told me this story.

There was a woman who was a regular at the yoga studio. Front-row type of person. There was a sub instructor and the class was starting out slower than usual—a lot of "connecting to the breath," and then some head rolling, finding your "center," that kind of thing. And this woman in the front row was *wigging out*. Exasperated sighs and eye rolls. Finally, the yoga instructor asked her, "Is something wrong?" She exploded, "Yes! I need to burn five hundred calories a day. So, can we get on with it?" And the yoga instructor responded, "Well, maybe if you sit still for a second, you'd realize why you eat five hundred calories more than you need each day."

Oh, SNAP.

That story bitch-slapped me so hard. Because I was just like that woman getting impatient in a yoga class. So resistant to drop my hustle. So not interested in doing the real work of sitting still and figuring myself out. Which is why I can totally empathize with my clients who come to me with patterns like this:

1. Run around like crazy all day.

2. Mindlessly eat whatever comes their way when they are
   ravenous because they don't have time to prepare.

3. Try to chill themselves out with wine at the end of the day.

And the cycle continues until they are burned-out and have a belly they can't get rid of.

This kind of high-stress, high-adrenalin lifestyle makes it almost impossible to get Healthy as Fuck.

But before you go and park it on a mountain to *om* away the rest of your days, let me clarify something about stress: stress isn't always bad. Workouts are stress. Learning a difficult new skill is stressful. If everything was easy, we wouldn't be forced to grow and get better.

Our bodies and psychology are amazing at dealing with acute stress like that. We release hormones that give us a quick burst of energy and shut down nonessential functions so we can do the important task at hand. We are brilliantly designed to handle this kind of acute "what doesn't kill you makes you stronger" stress.

What our bodies (and brains) are less good at dealing with is chronic stress. The ever-present feelings of always hustling to keep up. Of being defeated. Of constantly worrying about bills. When we are in a state of chronic stress, our bodies release fat into the bloodstream for energy. We don't use that energy, so it builds up as plaque, which increases our risk of heart disease. Chronic stress also causes our bodies to shuffle fat to our midsections in an effort to protect our vital organs from this perceived threat. Chronic stress leads to anxiety, depression, and sleep disorders, and then it increases our appetites and makes us crave sugar and fat.

So many of my clients are pushed to the limit and using snacks to make themselves feel better, to get a quick hit of energy or pleasure. For so many, that snack fiesta is probably the only fun thing that has happened to them all day. I'm telling you right now: if you don't allow yourself a little breathing space and a little fun, you will continue to reach for the snacks.

When people ask me, "What's more important, exercise or getting seven hours of sleep?" my answer is: "What's most important is designing a life that allows you to do both of these absolutely essential things without a trade-off.

When I say things like that, people think I don't understand that they have commitments and children and aging parents and jobs. I do get it. I promise I do. I've got all that stuff too. But before you repeat to me (and yourself) the story about how you are so busy, just remember that *you have a choice*. Even if you don't have a choice in your schedule (which you almost definitely do), you have a choice in the way you respond to that schedule.

What I mean is this: many people believe that they have to work long hours when really it's up to them to create clear boundaries for what they will and will not do. Many people believe it's necessary to have a big house, and entertain friends at a certain level of fanciness, and take their kids to karate lessons, and all the rest. I'm not saying any of this stuff is bad by any means. But they are *choices that you've made*. And if your choices are making you live a life of stress, then maybe it's time to rethink them.

Even if you don't want to reconsider the structures of your life, could you change your response? Is it possible to do it all with more ease and fun? Or does it have to be all duty and furrowed brows and high pressure? Does the morning routine really have to be so frantic, or can you add some playfulness? Would you maybe enjoy your hour-long commute in traffic if you listened to a wicked mystery novel while driving? What would the real impact be if you didn't check your email all weekend? Is your debt, your kids, your job really a life-or-death situation? Does stressing about it help at all? If you decided to take everything way less seriously and actually enjoy yourself more, would anything really collapse? As Mark Twain wrote: "I have known many sorrows, most of which never happened."

What's most important is designing a life that allows you to do both of these absolutely essential things without a trade-off.

I know that life is probably demanding a lot from you. But I'm telling you that creating some space and some joy in your life is essential. It's like when you are on a plane and they tell you to put the oxygen mask on yourself before you assist anyone else. If you have been playing the martyr and moaning about how you are so busy looking after other people, *stop it*. You've got to take care of yourself and your stress level—otherwise you are no good to anyone.

As your loving coach, I challenge you to come up with some ways you could simplify your life. Do you need to have a talk with your boss? Or tell your family to pick up some slack around the house? If you've got some cash to throw at this whole healthy living thing, it's totally possible that hiring a housekeeper is the best "weight loss/ health and wellness" dollars you will ever spend.

Once I was listening to a keynote speaker at a fitness conference with about twenty thousand fitness professionals. The speaker asked us to stand up if we felt like we were in good shape. Most of us stood up. And then he asked who ate only healthy food. There was some giggling as fewer people stood up this time. Then he asked who felt that their life was filled with happiness and joy. And guess what? Almost no one stood up. Like, crickets.

And I was like, wow. This is fucked. Everyone in this room needs to stop counting push-ups and carbs and start counting how often they laugh every day. Not just because it will lead to better quality of life, but because it's also a key health predictor.

In Dan Buettner's book *The Blue Zones*, he examines diverse geographic pockets where people live unusually long and healthy lives. He looks at Loma Linda in California, Okinawa in Japan, Sardinia in Italy, Ikaria in Greece, and the Nicoya Peninsula in Costa Rica. In each of these areas, there are an unusually high number of super centenarians—people who not only live to be one hundred years old, but do so while staying vital and kicking ass. The Blue Zones research is about trying to identify the common factors between these areas that

would seem to have very little in common. One of the key common-
alities between all the Blue Zones was low-stress living, with lots of
strong social and family connections, and a deep sense of purpose.

If getting Healthy as Fuck is important to you, reducing any chronic
stress in your life has got to be a priority. Like, an emergency. I know
you've got shit to do, but at the end of the day, you've got one life to
live, and I suggest you design it with intention, rather than just running
around like a crazy person, unconsciously snacking and then trying
to burn five hundred calories a day to make up for it. Which brings
us back to our keystone habit and one of the most effective ways to
reduce stress: meditate for twenty minutes every day.

Now don't panic. In order to meditate, you don't need to roll your
eyes to the back of your head and chant or anything. Just sit comfort-
ably and pick something minorly interesting to focus on—your breath,
a candle, some soft music, or nature sounds. And every time you catch
your mind wandering toward your to-do list, or what you want to
have for dinner, or who shot JR—just gently pull your attention back
to your point of focus.

Treat your brain like an adorable little puppy that wants to bounce
everywhere, but you lovingly bring it back to where it's supposed to be
every time. Be aware that pretty much no one is able to really stop their
mind from bouncing around like a retro '80s pinball machine and just
accept it. I've had clients who have said, "I can't meditate. My mind
just won't focus." I know. That's the point. That's like saying, "I can't
exercise. I get out of breath." But if you exercise with consistency, you

will eventually get less out of breath. And if you meditate consistently, you will find you are better able to focus. Slow and steady improvement is what we are looking for here. Remember that compound interest chart?

Even so, meditation can be a tough sell for my clients. I mean, these people hired me to help them get abs, not enlightenment. One of them pushed back with the totally understandable question: "What is the real value of adding twenty minutes of daily meditation to my life? The idea of sitting there and being unproductive stresses me out more than anything. Spending the twenty minutes feels like a waste of time."

Meditation is like a gym for your brain.

I get it. And you've probably already heard that meditation is awesome for you. The latest research is showing that it can reduce the inflammation caused by stress, decrease your blood pressure, help you sleep, reduce chronic pain, and improve your emotional health in almost every way.

But if you are mostly interested in how meditation helps you lose weight, maybe it helps to think of it this way: meditation is like a gym for your brain. And if you haven't got the memo yet, most of the heavy lifting when it comes to getting a crazy-hot body is actually going to be happening in your brain. It's a lot easier to sculpt your physique if you sculpt your brain first. Large-scale neuroimaging studies show that meditation will decrease activity in the amygdala, which is involved in stress and fear responses as well as anxiety. And it strengthens areas of the brain that are involved in emotional regulation, body awareness, and introspection. Which means that when you take the time to meditate every day:

- You are less likely to overeat. (Which is the primary reason people are overweight. More on that coming up.)
- You will be less likely to want alcohol to help you relax because you don't feel as stressed out.
- You will be more in tune with your body and connected to real hunger and satiety cues.
- You will improve your self-awareness, so you can recognize your triggers and also might get some insight on what might make you happy that isn't shoving gelato in your face.
- You promote self-compassion, which is critical for long-term success. Remember that negative, self-hating thoughts will lead to negative, self-hating behavior. Meditation is where you catch those unhelpful thoughts and blow them away like a fart in the breeze.

Developing that self-compassion is probably the most important benefit of meditation when it comes to getting Healthy as Fuck. Meditating every day will lead to a greater acceptance and love of exactly how your body is *right now*.

Which is, as we've already covered, the real objective. You just have to practice. And meditating will help.

HABIT #5: EAT IT ALL, BUT EAT *WAY* LESS OF IT

When I used to do one-on-one personal training, the first session with a new client would involve mostly talking. We'd sit down in their living room, I'd do a lifestyle interview, and we'd try to figure out why they weren't getting the results they wanted. They almost always thought it was an exercise problem...or a thyroid problem...or adrenal fatigue... or maybe just something that happens once you get older.

When I would ask about their diet, they would always say, "I eat really healthy!" And they did—these people were not trying to convince me that Pop-Tarts have fruit in them so they are healthy. They are people who spend top dollar on having a personal trainer come to their house. They are stone-cold serious about this shit.

And almost always, they are stone-cold overeating. They usually had no idea.

For instance, Tara reported that she was really "good"—she would always make herself a salad with some protein for dinner. She had young kids and they would have macaroni or whatever kid food, but Tara would have her salad with protein. This sounds great in theory, but here was the reality: While Tara was making food for her family, she was having bites and licks and tastes, along with a glass of wine. After dinner, she'd tidy up the dishes, and of course there's no point in saving those last few bites of ketchup-soaked macaroni, so she'd just eat the leftovers before putting the dishes in the dishwasher. And then when the kids went to bed, she'd make herself a little snack because, after all, she'd only had a salad for dinner. In reality, Tara had probably consumed two meals' worth of calories by the end of the night.

Let's take Barbara's story as another example. Barbara had previously seen temporary, but really promising, results with a paleo/keto/low-carb diet. So she had very strong ideas about certain foods being good (those with lots of protein and fat) and certain foods being bad (those that contained carbohydrates of any kind). By the time she hired me, Barbara was getting really frustrated because her weight was creeping up, even though she wasn't doing anything "bad." She was following the diet that had worked so well—she was avoiding all carbs! But she was also eating a fuck-ton of chicken breasts and sugar-free coconut bliss balls because according to her low-carb plan, they were "allowed" in unlimited amounts. Result: Barbara was tired, grumpy...and gaining weight.

Those are two examples of clients who believed they were eating "really healthy" but were still gaining weight. But most of my clients just overserve themselves. They eat beautiful, healthy food (I work with a lot of self-described "foodies")—but just way too much of it.

Here's an example: Nuts are really healthy, right? Absolutely—nuts are loaded with healthy fats that will lower your cholesterol, and they are an antioxidant powerhouse. But an appropriate serving is the size of your thumb—about eight almonds. Not a handful. Organic tofu is a great source of plant-based protein, but a serving would be the size of your palm. Oats are fantastic. A serving would be about the size of your fist (that's cooked, dude). Most people will easily eat twice these amounts.

I have so many clients who would tell me "I don't know why I can't lose weight—all I ever eat are salads." But their salads include half an avocado, plus dressing, plus a sprinkling of cheese, plus a boiled egg and some nuts. While it's awesome and huge high fives that they are eating such healthy, nutrient-dense food, there is just too much of it on that plate if fat reduction is part of their goals.

Maybe the examples sound familiar. Maybe you snack too much at work. Or have automatic second helpings. Or eat until you feel just a little bit too full. The fact is that if you have any of these unconscious habits of overeating, no matter how healthy the food is, it will lead to excess body fat.

You can't ignore good old fashioned CICO, which is fitness dork shorthand for Calories In, Calories Out. I know, no one talks about calories anymore. It's like you just stepped into a Tab cola commercial from the '80s. The trend for many years now has been to demonize a certain food or food group rather than talk about calories. This allows us to externalize the problem. The enemy is sugar! It's carbs that have done this to me! It's not that I'm eating too much. I can eat as much as I want as long as there aren't any carbs! Note: Telling people to eat less isn't going to make anyone any money, which is why it's not emphasized in popular culture. However, telling people that they need to avoid carbs will spawn a whole industry of low-carb alternative foods.

In telling people to eliminate carbohydrates (or whatever the latest baddy is), often a caloric deficit is created, and that initial weight loss will happen. Yay! However, eliminating any major macronutrient is unsustainable because it will result in intense cravings until you satisfy that need. Macronutrients are, by definition, nutrients that your body needs to survive—and you need to get them from food. Your body will send you signals to eat until that is fulfilled.

There have been studies showing that when given low-fat foods, subjects will consume 60 percent more calories. Why? Because they keep eating, trying to fulfill that need for adequate fat. Which is why you've got to eat carbs, protein, *and* fat. In a reasonable amount. No need to start tracking calories, because that's the worst way to spend your life with maximum head-fuck potential.

Here's the less bonkers plan.

Eat veggies! Fill half your plate with vegetables! ALL of them.

We've already covered this, but just to get you all pumped up again about the fat-blasting potential of this habit, remember that filling half your plate with veggies takes care of most of your CICO. It will fill you up with dietary fiber so you aren't hungry and pack you full of nutrients that will make you immortal. (Okay, not quite, but veggies are the closest thing we've got to the elixir of youth and vitality.) Great sources of veggies include: any of them. Anything leafy and colorful is awesome. Just try to avoid anything fried or swimming in sugary, fatty sauce.

Eat protein! Limit it to the size of your palm.

As I mentioned earlier, you really don't have to stress about meeting your protein requirements. Even if you do go 100 percent plant-based, you can easily meet your protein requirements as long as you are eating real food (versus vegan junk food, which totally exists—just because Doritos are vegan doesn't mean they are good for you, sorry).

Protein is a macronutrient that we need to live, and it's awesome for weight loss because it builds and repairs muscles and tissue. Maintaining your lean muscle mass (through working your muscles—this doesn't happen with protein alone) will increase your resting metabolic rate and facilitate a smokin' body composition. Protein also will help you feel full longer, as it takes longer to digest than carbs. An appropriate portion of protein would be the size of your palm (both diameter and thickness), and the best choices would be legumes, tofu, and tempeh; remember that the conclusions of the China Study were to eat as much plant-based foods as possible and avoid animal products for maximum health and longevity. Next-best options would be wild-caught fish, poultry, and free-range eggs. Even lean red meat should be limited due to its association with earlier mortality and heart disease.

SERIOUSLY AVOID: processed meat and deli slices and fatty meat like bacon.

Eat carbs! Limit them to the size of your fist.

Hell yeah, you can eat carbs and get lean and healthy! In fact, you kind of have to.

Carbohydrates are the primary energy source for your body and your brain. If you don't eat carbs, you will have low energy and be kind of dumb.

Remember those Orange People I used to certify as personal

trainers? Sometimes I'd be teaching them while they were in the final stages of their "cut" phase, which is when they build a ton of muscle by eating a lot and doing a lot of strength training, and then they "cut" the fat on top of the muscle by going on a strict low-fat, low-carb diet and doing HIIT cardio training. It ends up looking hot as hell, and I know it's tempting to just drop this book and follow their lead to get to the same look, but just a reminder: none of them looked that way in real life because it's impossible to sustain.

So this fitness competitor came to my personal training course, about a week before his competition. He brought a BUCKET of cooked ground beef to my course and just spent all day eating it with a spoon, right out of the bucket. Not only was he lacking somewhat in dining decorum, but he also kept apologizing for not understanding the material and explained that he hadn't eaten any carbs in a week, so he was feeling a bit mentally foggy.

Point being: you need carbs to function. There is nothing wrong with carbs. However, not all carbs are created equal. This might look like a low-carb program to you, but it's really more of a *smart-carb* program.

Great carbs: sweet potatoes, beets, legumes (yes, beans and legumes are a carb and a protein; don't stress about it—just eat them because they are a power food, loaded with B vitamins and fiber), potatoes, yams, squash, whole-grain rice, amaranth, oats, quinoa, buckwheat, all fruit

Bullshit carbs: highly processed carbs, such as white bread, pastries, crackers, anything with added sugar

Wait. Are you saying I can eat *bread*?

Well, I mean it would be great if all your carbs were unprocessed whole foods. But bread is a cultural staple for a lot of people, and there are bread options that would be a good source of carbs. Sprouted bread, whole-grain rye bread…these are awesome! But remember the portion should be one slice. So yes, I am saying that tofu/egg scramble with tons of veggies on a slice of whole-grain toast would be a great five-minute healthy meal. A sandwich with bologna and two slices of Wonder Bread is really…not.

What about sugar? It's the devil, right?

I don't think sugar is necessarily the devil, and recent comparisons to cocaine are probably a little exaggerated. Again, it's a portion control thing. The WHO recommends that sugar account for no more than 5 percent of our caloric intake, or about six teaspoons a day. That sounds like a lot until you consider that includes added sugars or naturally occurring sugars in juice or natural sweeteners like honey. The average North American gets three times that amount each day, and no wonder. Sugar is added to everything these days. Your ready-made coleslaw, your frozen pizza, your orange-chicken glaze, your yogurt, your onion soup. There is more sugar in your ketchup than there is in vanilla ice cream.

The easiest way for you to avoid sugar is to make your own food from real whole food sources as described here.

That way, you can save your six teaspoons of sugar for something that's worth it (like a square or two of dark chocolate) instead of getting punked when your tomato sauce puts you over the limit, spiking your blood sugar and making you hungry a few hours later. If you are currently in the habit of drinking sweetened drinks like soda or iced tea—quit it. That is a bunch of liquid nonsense that is making you fat and unhealthy. I don't care if it's got zero calories; those fake sugar substitutes are associated with cancer and are just training your palate to want more sweet, chemical bullshit. Switch to water and watch your waist get smaller and your health get better. If you really love flavored drinks, there are some herbal teas that are so delicious they should be illegal.

Eat fat! Limit it to the size of your thumb.

Why? Fat is a major source of energy, transports certain vitamins, is essential for cellular health, and makes you feel satisfied.

- **Awesome fats:** nuts and seeds (flax, sesame, chia), avocado, olives, nut butters
- **Less awesome:** dairy fat (cheese, yogurt, milk, cream), animal fats (lard, fatty meat like bacon)

AVOID LIKE THE PLAGUE: Trans fats. These are found in vegetable shortening, some margarine, baked goods and crackers, fried foods,

and anything that lists "partially hydrogenated oils." Remember how
I said eating a shit-ton of vegetables was basically the only thing that
everyone agrees on when it comes to nutrition? Just kidding, I lied.
Not eating any trans fats is the other thing. Even small amounts of
trans fats can fuck you over: even a 2 percent increase of calories from
trans fats has been associated with a 34 percent increase in all-cause
mortality. The best way to avoid this stuff is to stop buying processed
foods. Instead, make your own damn cookies from scratch. Don't buy
the ones on the shelf. There's a reason they stay fresh on the shelf for
months, and that's because trans fats have been added to keep them
stabilized. A good rule of thumb thrown around by dieticians is: if your
food can't go bad, it's not good for you.

Okay, you've got the trans-fat thing, but did you get that fat
portion recommendation? One thumb-sized portion of healthy fats.
This is where you might be looking at your adorable little thumb and
thinking, *Wait a second. THAT is all the peanut butter I get?! I'm
clearly going to starve.*

Let me assure you that you will not starve. When you eat quality
food and tons of high-fiber, nutrient-dense veggies instead of sugar and
processed carbs, you will find that you are satisfied with less. When you
eat appropriate amounts of all the macronutrients instead of depriving
yourself of an entire category of food that you need to live, you'll find
that you have fewer cravings.

Here are some other tips to help you reset your appetite and eat
less.

Don't eat unless you are genuinely hungry.

Duh, right? Except a lot of us really suck at that, especially in North America. Some cultures have got it figured out: In Okinawa, Japan, it is customary to say *hara hachi bun me* ("eat until the belly is 80 percent full") before every meal. This gastronomic restraint probably contributes to Okinawans' relatively low BMIs, which is thought to be one of the reasons why Okinawa is one of the Blue Zones of exceptional longevity.

The Ayurvedic tradition from India is one of the world's oldest holistic healing practices and recommends eating until 75 percent full. And in France (a culture known for being inexplicably thin despite huffing back croissants like no one's business), they don't say, "I'm full" after a meal. They say, "I'm no longer hungry."

This is what you want to aim for when eating: no longer hungry. It's time to stop riding the standard North American cycle of stuffed and starving. Here's how you do it.

Slow. The. Fuck. Down.

This is another one of those ways that mindfulness and generally chilling the fuck out is really the key to losing weight. If you eat in a distracted way or shovel it in between activities like there's a prize for first place, you are not giving your body any opportunity to tell you that you've had enough.

The challenge I'm going to give you is to spend twenty minutes eating each meal. Bonus points if you eat that meal without any distractions (computer, TV, book). Put down your fork between bites. Chew. Breathe. Drink a sip of water. Think about what you are doing instead of wondering five minutes later what black magic fuckery made your burrito disappear. Consider how you like the food. Have the balls to go off autopilot for the twenty minutes it takes to eat your meal and allow your inner wisdom to shine through with profound insights like "Holy fuck. I actually don't feel like I need this entire burrito after all."

Know the difference between genuine hunger and a craving.

Here's the deal:

- Cravings will go away if you distract yourself or wait them out. Hunger will return no matter what.
- Cravings will usually be for a specific kind of food. If you are hungry, broccoli looks good. If you aren't hungry for vegetables, you aren't hungry.
- Cravings are usually emotionally or situationally driven. Hunger is physical. You feel it in your stomach, or sometimes it feels like a headache or light-headedness.

The thing is that most of us give into our cravings so much that we don't even know what hunger feels like.

If you aren't hungry for vegetables, you aren't hungry.

Experience hunger.

There's a good chance you rarely experience hunger. Kids these days are basically on an IV drip of Goldfish crackers. Even health-minded adults will graze all day under the pretense of keeping their metabolisms revved.

Allow yourself to get hungry and then *don't panic*. Hunger isn't an emergency. Diarrhea is an emergency. Tell yourself you can have food anytime you want, but you just want to experience being hungry for a few minutes.

Hunger isn't an emergency. Diarrhea is an emergency.

Once you get to know real hunger, you will start to become better acquainted with how it feels in your body versus a craving. What you think is genuine hunger may actually be your body's conditioned response to your accustomed pattern of eating (your habit). If you interrupt that habit, you can reset the pattern. Even if you *are* actually physically hungry, remember that no one has ever died of starvation between lunch and dinner. You will be okay. I get that you might hate the feeling of being hungry, but know that it's your emotions that hate the feeling—your body is just fine. After adapting for centuries of food scarcity, your body knows how to deal with being hungry. When not getting its usual number of calories, the body says, "I know! Let's metabolize stored energy!"

On the other hand, our bodies have not yet evolved to handle excess amounts of food. Our system gets overloaded trying to digest and process the overwhelming amount of food, and it uses up a lot of energy and makes us grumpy. (That's why you want to go to sleep after your Thanksgiving meal, by the way. It's not the tryptophan. There is just as much tryptophan in nuts and cheese as turkey.)

BONUS: Allowing genuine hunger before your meals will also make your food taste crazy delicious.

In conclusion, eat it all! Protein, carbohydrates, and fats are all essential to live, and none of them are "bad." Enough with the macronutrient witch-hunt silliness. Just eat whole, unprocessed foods and keep to the portion sizes recommended here. If you follow this simple plan, you will easily shed extra fat, feel so much more energy, and increase your chances of living a long and healthy life. I'm not shitting you when I say that food is powerful medicine. But just like any medicine, *there is an optimal dose*. An apple a day keeps the doctor away. But forty-three apples a day will make you gain weight and give you nasty farts.

And just so you don't end up in a situation where you are tempted to eat forty-three apples in a day, you might want to start doing Healthy Habit #6...

HABIT #6: PREP AND PLAN AHEAD

Pop quiz: What is the number-one reason people give when asked why they aren't in good shape? You got it: "I don't have the time."

Unfortunately, we have to admit that this is bullshit in so many ways. And I'm not even talking about the fact that most of the people who say that have probably found the time to binge-watch something on Netflix or get into a heated fight with someone in the comments section on the internet. It's bullshit because *making a healthy choice usually doesn't take more time.* Let me explain with an example.

My friend Laura said to me, "I've really been trying to eat healthy, but the other day was so busy that I wanted something quick and I just threw a frozen pizza in the oven."

This is a scenario we can all relate to, but it actually makes no logical sense. A frozen pizza takes about twenty minutes to cook. And that's after the oven preheats (which takes approximately five lifetimes when you are hungry). Some chickpeas sautéed with a couple of handfuls of fresh spinach and one tablespoon of delicious pesto takes about three minutes. The problem is not that Laura didn't have the time; it's that she was stressed out after a busy day, so she unconsciously executed her stress habit loop (trigger = stress, behavior = eat pizza, reward = brain releases endorphins as a response to salty, fatty food and feeling of "treating" herself).

We don't need more time—we need better habits.

When people say they don't have time to get in shape, they imagine commuting to a gym for an hour-long workout every day and then battling traffic to come home and start wrestling with a butternut squash and marinating some protein when everyone is starving and grumpy and wanting dinner like, yesterday. I agree. For most of us, that is a fucking nightmare. Because most of us do feel strapped for time. So, if this Healthy as Fuck project is gonna happen, it needs to happen in the most time-efficient way possible.

Introducing: the Meal Prep Power Hour. If you want to lose body fat and get 'er done with the least amount of time spent, then you need to allocate some time each week toward prepping healthy food. *This is the absolute most efficient use of your time if you want to lose weight.* If you are someone who has been working out every single day but you are experiencing a weight-loss plateau, I challenge you to skip one of your workouts and use the time to do my Meal Prep Power Hour—and watch your body shrink.

We don't need more time— we need better habits.

Here's why: If you have good food in your fridge, you will eat good food. If you don't make the effort to have good food in your fridge, you will eat according to your current habit pattern, which is resulting in your current body. Which very well might be a totally awesome and slammin' body, but if you've read this far, I'm assuming that losing some fat is important to you. And if losing some fat is important to you, then it's going to be all about changing your diet.

Yes, exercising is totally important as well, and I'll explain that in the next habit. But if weight loss is your primary goal and you are strapped for time, it is WAY more efficient to not eat those calories in the first place than to try to "work them off" with exercise. And the best way to ensure that you will eat healthy, nutrient-dense food with a low caloric load is to prep and plan in advance.

Seriously, dude. Don't fall into the trap of thinking that this healthy eating shit is just going to happen on its own. Just have a look at how many veggies are available at your local Starbucks, where people think the "healthy" option is getting a soy latte with some sugar-free bullshit syrup because it's low carb. Look around at how fat and tired and unhealthy almost everyone is, and you will realize that if you want to look and feel different from the rest of the world, you will have to act different from the rest of the world. "Going with the flow" is deciding to be out of shape and unhealthy. Period. You cannot rely on good food being available to you. You need to plan in advance and make it happen. It's not as hard as you think, and it is the best investment of time you can give toward your healthy and hot bod.

Here's a sample Meal Prep Power Hour. I do something like this every Sunday to set me up for healthy lunches, easy dinners, and healthy snacks. If you want a Meal Prep Power Hour that includes specific recipes, grab it at www.fitfeelsgood.com/book.

This sample menu includes:

- Roasted veggies
- Quinoa
- Hummus + veggies

- Salad bar + dressing
- Prepped protein
- Power balls

Set your timer for one hour.

READY...

SET...

PREP!

Step #1: Roast your veggies.

If the thought of filling half of every plate with raw veggies makes you want to cry, you'll definitely want to have some roasted veggies on hand. It completely changes the texture of the vegetables and often brings out their natural sweetness. You'll want to include some of the allium family (onions, garlic, etc.) here, which are not easy to eat raw but have powerful antioxidants and give lots of natural flavor to your food without adding calories. Peppers, zucchini, and root vegetables like parsnips and sweet potatoes are all awesome roasting options as well.

Once you have roasted veggies on hand for the week you can put them on a salad, add them to a sandwich, puree them into a soup, or add them to a grain bowl. The party never stops.

Preheat oven to about 400°F; wash and chop veggies; toss with a little bit of olive oil, salt, and pepper; and throw them in the oven. Set your alarm to check on them every twenty minutes or so, and remove when you see the toasty bits happening.

Step #2: Get quinoa (or some other grain) cooking.

You want to switch up your grain choice every week for maximum nutritional diversity, but the reason quinoa is such a big deal is because it's not actually a grain—it's a seed. (That's why it looks like it "sprouts" when you cook it.) This means that it has a lower glycemic index, is higher in protein *and* fiber, and contains awesome, hard-to-get nutrients like magnesium. It's also gluten-free, if that's a thing for you (*wink*).

You can use your cooked quinoa as a yummy breakfast option that's high in plant-based protein: heat it up with some cinnamon, add some almond milk, and top with some fruit and nuts. You can toss some quinoa in your salad to make it more filling. Or make a quick grain bowl for dinner by adding some roasted veggies and pesto.

Step #3: Getcher hummus on.

I know there are thirty varieties of hummus at your grocery store, but chances are that they are all made with some nasty cheap oil, so you are missing a chance to absorb some of the good, anti-inflammatory fats you would find in good-quality olive oil. Not a bad idea to switch up your legumes and make a black bean spread or whatever next week. Hummus is just some chickpeas, tahini, olive oil, and lemon juice in a food processor. Chuck in some spices and let your creativity soar. You are now an artist whose medium is bean dip.

Or, if you are brave, give your kid a potato masher and let them smush it all up while you get on with your life.

Step #4: Salad bar time!

I know, I know. You don't win friends with salad. The trick is to make it as varied and delicious as possible, so you don't feel sad about your life every time you pull out your lunch at work.

Make sure you have a selection of salad toppings that you love. Think avocado, seeds, olives, some cheese if you are down with dairy. (The fat from cheese isn't as good as the fat from the others, but hey, if it's the spoonful of sugar that helps the medicine go down, that's cool.)

Buy a selection of greens (whatever works—just switch it up every week or so). If not prewashed, then tear it up into bite-sized bits, wash it, dry it, and package it. Chop up a shit-ton of veggies: peppers, carrots, celery, cucumber (bonus points for seasonal), and portion it out into mason jars or containers for quick grab-and-go ability. Make sure to cut some vegetables in sticks for hummus dipping.

Step #5: Make your own dressing.

It is not easy to find salad dressing at the grocery store that isn't full of cheap oils and weird shit. Skip it and make one at home with oil and vinegar instead. This is your chance to use up that fancy flavored vinegar that someone gave you for Christmas two years ago. The classic ratio is one part vinegar to three parts oil. Add some herbs, crushed garlic, and mustard for some tang, and shake it all up in a container that seals tight. This formula tastes so much better than commercial salad dressing that you will be overreacting to your salad like you are auditioning for a stock photographer.

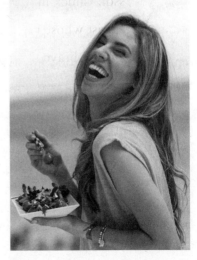

Step #6: Prep some protein.

By now the quinoa should be done, so you can put that away in the fridge (seal it up tight: should last three to five days) and use the same pot to make some red lentils. Lentils are a great source of iron and folate, and if you've got cooked lentils on hand, they can be added to bulk up a salad, smushed into a patty for a quick veggie burger, folded into a whole grain (or lettuce) wrap for a taco-type thing or added to a soup to make it more of a meal. I do one cup of red lentils to two cups of veggie stock and let it simmer for about fifteen minutes.

If lentils aren't your jam, you could also whip up a marinade in a container and throw some chopped tofu (or your protein of choice) in there. Tofu on its own tastes pretty bland, but it's great because it will soak up any marinade and be a little protein-packed flavor bomb that you can throw on your veggies without even having to cook it first.

Step #7: Make some power balls.

I will often get asked which are the best bars to have around in case of emergency. It's a good question because a lot of us eat on the go and most of the "nutrition" bars on the market are about as good for you as an Oh Henry! bar. Homemade power balls are easy and way healthier than the shitty protein bars you are currently eating. If you are trying to lose weight, I'd recommend you keep your snacks to vegetables—or fruit if you want something sweet. However, on days when that's just not going to cut it, you can make your own power balls. These will keep you going and satisfy your need for a treat while packing in some healthier slow-release energy.

While the lentils are cooking, wash the food processor well (you don't want your power balls to taste like garlic from the hummus). Throw in two parts oats to one part nut butter (tahini for a nut-free, school-safe alternative), a splash of maple syrup or honey, and then get wild with add-ins like flax and sesame seeds, hemp hearts, shredded coconut, raisins, or dark chocolate chips. Play with flavors like cinnamon, cacao, or vanilla and switch it up each week.

Pulse until it all clumps together. Roll into small balls (this is another great "What a big helper you are!" project for kids) and store in the fridge for a quick hit of energy preworkout.

Step #8: Package and clean up!

By this point, the lentils and the roasted veggies should be done. Let them both cool on the counter to room temperature before you package them up in sealed containers. The veggies should last three to five days, and you

> Pick your battles and remember that none of this shit has to be perfect.

might get a whole week out of the lentils. Glass and stainless-steel containers are ideal, but I'll be honest and say I still have some plastic floating around. Pick your battles and remember that none of this shit has to be perfect. Every little step in the right direction counts.

Step #9: Celebrate!

Once everything is stored in the fridge, kick back and relax with the satisfaction that you just spent a very productive hour toward getting Healthy as Fuck.

HABIT #7: EXERCISE CONSISTENTLY

The other day, my client Sarah said something that broke my heart and made me realize that maybe I've been one of those asshole trainers. Here's what happened.

She posted in our group: "Oonagh, is Zumba the same as your quad workout?"

I wrote back: "Zumba would be a great replacement for something like a run because it's endurance cardio. My quad workout is strength training and high-intensity interval training (HIIT), which works different energy systems and is more efficient for weight loss."

I shouldn't have said it.

Now, don't get me wrong—this is all totally true. The best type of exercise to lose weight in the shortest amount of time is to do strength training and HIIT. HIIT is a type of cardio training in which you just go balls-out hard for a short period of time and then rest and then do it again. The other type of cardio training is LISS, which stands for Low-Intensity Steady State. HIIT would be doing a hundred-meter sprint and resting and doing it again for about twenty minutes. LISS would be going for a forty-minute easy jog.

Trainers love HIIT because you can get the same fat-burning results with less time spent exercising. If you have ever thought to yourself, *If only I had a trainer, then I would know the real secret magic to getting super fit*—I'll just tell you right now, there is no secret magic. If you want to lose body fat, most trainers today will eventually get you doing strength training and HIIT. It's important to note that I said *eventually*. Before you even *think* about the "best" way to train, you need to get consistent. Developing a regular routine that you stick to is about a million gazillion times more important than the type of exercise you do.

That's where I fucked up. Because Sarah wrote back: "Oh, I'm so mad at myself! I thought I had done something good."

SHIT.

Sarah had never really been able to get her exercise habit off the ground, and she finally found something she liked, and I made her feel like it was "wrong." The only appropriate answer here would have been: "You tried a Zumba class? You are awesome! When is the next one?"

Instead, I behaved like one of those douche-bag trainers who comes up to you in the gym and tells you that you are squatting all wrong and you'll probably hurt your knees so you should probably pay him $3,000 to awkwardly watch you squat for the next year as it's the only way to prevent a total nuclear meltdown of your body.

That is the kind of bullshit that keeps people scared of exercise or feeling like they shouldn't bother if they can't do it "right." All this concern about proper form is over-exaggerated and hardly necessary for people who are mostly moving their own body weight. Seriously. Anyone who tells you that you are "doing it wrong" is trying to sell you something.

Here's how you check your own form:

1. Am I moving?
2. Am I pain-free?

If you answered yes to the previous two questions, your form is a hell of a lot better than everyone parked on the couch watching TV right now.

Now maybe you are thinking, *Wait a second, Oonagh. Isn't it supposed to hurt a little?*

No. Repeat after me: "Exercise should never hurt."

Will it always feel comfortable?

Fuck no.

If you are comfortable, you aren't challenging yourself. By the end of a set of push-ups, your muscles should be begging for mercy. But that's not pain. Pain is caused by an illness or injury, and it's not a normal experience of exercise.

It's understandable that new exercisers get confused when we've all been fed the "no pain, no gain" line since Jane Fonda first donned a pair of leg warmers. I actually had a client once who was so out of shape she didn't even like casual walking. I started her training program slowly by asking her to clap her hands over her head while sitting down. She started and then immediately protested, "It hurts! It hurts!" I was completely baffled until I realized that when she said, "It hurts," she just meant that she was experiencing exercise-induced muscle fatigue by lifting her arms up and she freaking hated that feeling.

So, here's how you tell whether you are experiencing the good I'm-challenging-myself-and-getting-stronger *discomfort* vs. the bad holy-fuck-don't-do-that-ever-again *pain*.

> **"Challenging myself" discomfort:** Usually feels like a gradual onset of a burning type of sensation that you feel right in the muscle (not the joint). The feeling will go away when you stop doing the movement.

> **"Oh shit, something went wrong" pain:** Usually a sudden, sharp pain, often felt near the joint, that will result in you not wanting to use that part of your body, even after the exercise is over.

Got it? Great. You are ready to exercise. Seriously.

Off you go now.

What are you waiting for?

Oh—are you waiting to have more free time? Do you really think there is ever going to come a moment when all your emails are answered and the house is spotless with the laundry all folded and your kids want nothing to do with you and you are going to look around and shrug your shoulders and think, *Well, I've got some time on my hands. Guess I might as well do some exercise now?* That moment won't happen. There will always be more important things to do if you don't put this first. And if you don't put exercising first, you will lose functioning of your body and your life will seriously suck. If you don't use it, you lose it. Your amazingly efficient body will start to atrophy those muscles, and then you won't be able to use them when you want to, for stuff like stairs. Like tying your shoes. Like getting off a toilet without assistance. Seriously, who wants help getting off a toilet? No one. Make the time to exercise. There is no excuse. And just a reminder, your heart is a muscle. If you don't use it (by raising your heart rate), then it will also lose function. Also known as dying. And no one wants that either.

You can't wait until you have "more time." And no, you don't need more money either. Take Oprah. Remember Marathon-Running Oprah? It was after Wagon-of-Fat Oprah, but before Spiritual Oprah. Anyway, Marathon-Running Oprah was talking about her new fitness kick, and somebody challenged her and said, "Yeah, I could get in shape, too, if I had money for a personal trainer and a personal chef!"

To which Marathon-Running Oprah apparently responded: "I can have all the personal trainers in the world, but it's my fat ass that's running around that track."

Point being: your personal fitness is the one thing you can't outsource. Otherwise I'm sure Oprah would have. Yes, you throw some money at it and get some help and that is awesome. I'm so proud to say that is exactly what I do for a living. *But you still need to take radical responsibility for your results.* I have the lovely experience of receiving almost daily emails from people saying, "Thank you so much! Because of you, I've lost weight and totally changed my life and I feel incredible!" And although I love getting those emails and they fill my heart with joy, I always counter: "I didn't do a single one of your planks. I didn't eat salad when I wanted a chimichanga. YOU did that. Those results happened because of your actions, not mine." On the other hand, I will occasionally get an email that says something along the lines of "I bought your program and it didn't work!" And then when I ask them if they actually *did* the program after purchasing it, the answer is "Well, no…" (Seriously, this happens.) Because people are desperately looking to outsource responsibility for their health, but it just doesn't work that way.

At the end of the day, you just need to get up and do it. You don't need more money. Push-ups, crunches, and running are free. And the internet is a tickle trunk of free workouts as well. (If you want my curated list of the best Free Fitness on the web, go to www.fitfeelsgood.com/book.)

Just do something. Pretty much every day. Even on your vacation. Even on days when you don't fucking feel like it. ("Yoga for When You Are Hungover" is one of the links on my Free Fitness resources. You're welcome.) It doesn't have to be hard—start with a walk around the block. It doesn't have to be long—my clients and I do a twenty-minute strength and HIIT training program, and we are so ripped and hot, it's crazy. It just has to happen consistently. No negotiations. No hitting the Snooze button and then lying there having a big, old debate about whether you REALLY have to exercise today because *blah blah insert-excuse-here blah*. Or trying to make a deal with yourself about how you'll exercise later or skip a meal to make up for it. Listen to how funny your brain is trying to wiggle out of it and then get the fuck up and exercise anyway. (More about this when we "Break Up with Your Bullshit" in chapter 8.) It can be anything as long as you are moving. Step outside the box and think about what movement you might genuinely look forward to. What did you love doing when you were a kid? Swimming? Skating? Climbing? Find something you love—or at least something you don't hate—and go for it.

When people ask me, "What is the best exercise?" I know they are looking for my educated trainer answer (which would be the standard "strength training and HIIT cardio" if they are looking to lose fat), but really I want to tell them to just put on their favorite music and dance like a fool and laugh and have fun. Because if you are having fun, you will actually DO it. At this point of my life, I think that strength training and HIIT cardio is more fun than tequila shots and a sombrero, but that certainly wasn't always the case. Remember that in order to get consistent I had to bribe myself with trashy, guilty pleasure TV.

> Listen to how funny your brain is trying to wiggle out of it and then get the fuck up and exercise anyway.

So, if you aren't yet exercising consistently, what do you need to do to make that happen? You need to take radical responsibility for your health and figure out what would be fun or at least tolerable enough that you would commit for real.

The idea is to move you up this continuum:

At the bottom, we have Sedentary Sally. She drives to work, sits at a desk, drives home, and then sits and watches TV. This is pretty common and why most North Americans get only about five thousand steps a day (versus the ten thousand recommended for adults).

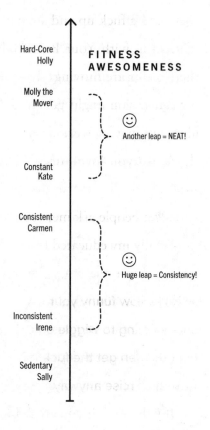

Just above that we have Inconsistent Irene. She exercises sometimes, but she can't get that consistency down. She will get a burst of motivation and maybe work out three times in one week, but then the next week is a write-off. And she manages one the week after, and then she gets sick, etc., etc. (Don't get me wrong, Irene is doing WAY better than Sally! She's broken the seal—that is a huge accomplishment! But as far as seeing any difference in the way she looks and feels, she's probably going to experience going one step forward, one step back, and get seriously frustrated.)

Then there is Consistent Carmen, who goes to a dance or yoga or rock-climbing class three times a week. If she's happy with her results, then I'm happy! However, if she wants to get leaner and healthier, I'd encourage her to increase her frequency or maybe join Kate...

Constant Kate goes to boot-camp class three times a week, where she does HIIT cardio and strength training. In doing so, she's being really efficient in revving up her metabolism and building lean muscle mass, therefore changing her body composition in the least amount of time.

But then there is Molly the Mover. She doesn't go to a gym or anything, but she's a farmer or a chef and she is moving all day every day and uses her muscles. She's lean, and her body functions really well. Physically, she seems much younger than her years. She really earns her Netflix at the end of the day.

Finally, there is Hard-Core Holly. Holly is working out most days a week where she works her muscles hard and gets out of breath and sweaty. She also bikes to work, goes for a walk on her lunch break, and does active play with her kids when she gets home, easily getting at least ten thousand steps a day. Holly is definitely above average in her fitness. She has tons of energy and looks hella tight.

(By the way, if you are reading this and thinking, *But I am a Hard-Core Holly! And I'm not hella tight, WTF?!*, then you are awesome because you've nailed this critical habit of consistently challenging your body to get stronger. The secret to busting your plateau is going to be in one of the other habits.)

Notice that the big leap was between Inconsistent Irene and Consistent Carmen. Notice the next big leap was between Constant Kate and Molly the Mover. You might be surprised because Molly doesn't work out, but she is leveraging NEAT (Non-Exercise Activity Thermogenesis), which is basically a fancy way of saying that she keeps her metabolism revved up

all day long and therefore has an elevated caloric burn all day long. The latest science shows that NEAT is one of the most underrated components of wellness. It basically means you just can't sit all day. It's fucking awful for you. It's way healthier to be on your feet and moving throughout the day than go balls-out at a spin class and then sit on your butt for the other twenty-three hours of the day. I tell all my clients to aim for ten thousand steps a day, get up and move every hour in order to counteract the effects of sitting, and get that NEAT revved up all day.

As your habits develop and you move up this continuum of exercise behavior, you will see why exercising consistently is one of the most powerful keystone habits you can implement for your life. You will see that you are less likely to eat Toaster Strudels for breakfast when you just came back from a run. Even if it was a pathetically slow ten-minute run. You will notice that you are less likely to kill half a bottle of wine every night if you are committed to going to boot camp in the morning. And that's just the immediate aftereffects of movement, not to mention the long-term health benefits of regular exercise.

When you exercise regularly, you will:

- Sleep better.
- Increase your energy.
- Reduce the risk of dementia.
- Improve your bone strength.
- Reduce your risk of a gazillion chronic diseases.
- Help your skin stay healthy and younger-looking.

- Have better sex (seriously—good cardiovascular health helps the blood flow *everywhere*).
- Reduce depression.
- Not DIE.

Did you, um, notice that losing weight isn't listed here? Surprise! Exercising certainly won't hurt your weight-loss attempts, but trying to burn off calories through exercise is actually a piss-poor weight-loss strategy. For example, to burn off a side order of fries, an average-sized person would have to go on the elliptical for about two hours. Unless you want to waste your life on an elliptical machine, it's way more efficient to just not eat the fries in the first place.

The idea of "burning off" food is an old-school mentality that doesn't work. Worse, it creates a head fuck where you start thinking things like *I did a hard workout so I deserve this treat* or *I'll order pizza tonight and just do a really hard workout tomorrow*. This leads to a "binge and purge" mentality that will:

1. Make you crazy.
2. Blow out your knees as you overexercise to burn off food.
3. Keep you fat because it doesn't work.

The role of exercise with fat loss is a bit more subtle. When you increase your lean muscle mass, you will have an elevated resting metabolism (because all those sexy muscles burn more calories when

you are just sitting around scrolling on Facebook). That's why trainers are always trying to get you to lift weights and build muscle, especially as you get older and muscle mass naturally declines with age. And no, it won't make you bulky, for fuck's sake—it will make you a total babe. In fact, in a study done by the Harvard School of Public Health, it was determined that the most effective training program for belly fat reduction for older adults was strength training for twenty minutes a day along with aerobic training. Any old aerobic training is great (go Zumba!), but if you want maximum results for the minimum amount of time in the gym, HIIT is the way to go. When you do HIIT and strength training, you are boosting your resting energy expenditure for up to seventy-two hours after the workout as your body recovers. What that means is that three days after you got your pump on you are still torching calories.

So that's why I answered Sarah the way I did when she asked me if Zumba was the same thing as my quad workout. It just isn't. But it was still kind of a dick answer for me to give because Sarah was at the Inconsistent Irene stage of things, and I made it sound like she fucked up by not being a full-out Hard-Core Holly. That would be like saying that someone who just ran their first marathon wasn't doing a good thing because she didn't win the race.

And just because exercise isn't the most important piece of the puzzle for weight loss doesn't mean you should dismiss it, even if eliminating your love handles is your primary goal. You remember how 99 percent of people who lose weight will gain it back? Guess what the other 1 percent do? They exercise. Do you remember that crushing article where they followed up with all *The Biggest Loser* contestants and they had mostly gained the weight back? Those who didn't *were the ones who had maintained a regular exercise routine.*

Just get into it. I know it can suck to start. Believe me, I spent the first half of my life avoiding exercise like it was E. coli. But let me tell you from the other side of the first awkward shuffling and gasping attempts—the cumulative effects of being a consistent exerciser are unbelievable. If Pfizer could package a pill that does everything that regular exercise does for you, it would be a total mic-drop moment for Big Pharma.

And here's the best part: you don't have to wait around to not have a heart attack in twenty years in order to be glad you exercised. You will notice the effects *immediately.*

What's not to love about that? It gives you the most immediate return on your time investment. Where else can you get that sweet-ass deal? As soon as you finish exercising, you will experience the natural exercise-induced endorphins that will make you feel happier and more relaxed and confident.

And might I remind you, feeling happy and relaxed and confident is actually our end goal. So if you are going to "skip to the end" and bask in happiness as I advised you to do when you got your head out of your ass in part 1, I suggest you get exercising. Now.

Oh, and by the way—if you've done the whole "Let's get fit!" New Year's resolution thing before…and by February all you've got to show for it is a ThighMaster gathering dust under your bed, never fear. Next, I'm going to tell you everything you need to know about How Not to Be a Big, Fat Quitty McQuitterface.

· PART 3 ·

HOW NOT TO BE A BIG, FAT QUITTY McQUITTERFACE

DO. OR DO NOT.
THERE IS NO TRY.

SO, ARE YOU EXCITED TO IMPLEMENT ALL 7 HABITS OF HIGHLY Healthy Motherfuckers?!

I hope this feels like a relief to know that what you need to do to get lean and healthy is actually much more simple than we are led to believe. You now have the keystone habits that are going to get you better results than all the brain clutter, clickbait bullshit that we are all subjected to every day. Never mind all the diet fads. These habits are the 20 percent effort that will give you 80 percent of your results.

If you start:

filling half your plate with vegetables,

getting at least seven hours of sleep,

ditching the booze,

eating appropriate portions,

prepping your food in advance,

chilling your ass out and meditating regularly, and

exercising consistently,

you will feel like a total babe, be Healthy as Fuck, and change pretty much your entire world—because you'll probably be a hell of a lot happier.

Which is, again, the actual point.

Yes, I know I keep hammering that home. But I'd be gutted if your takeaway from this book was "Oonagh said I'm not allowed to eat cheese anymore and Zumba is bad." So, let's review what we've covered so far so we are all on the same page of health and hotness:

1. In part 1, we talked about how you get to choose whether you actually want to lose weight. You understand that there is an effort-to-results ratio, and you get to choose what level of effort you want to give depending on what level of fitness you want to have. It's totally legit to tell six-pack abs to go fuck themselves, and it's also totally legit to decide that it's a goal that you want to achieve. Either way, you've got to know that it's not actually abs you are chasing, but the feeling you think you will have when you have the abs. That is, happiness. And the only way to get the happiness you want is to practice that feeling right now, at exactly the

weight you are at. Remember, the feeling is the actual goal, so we have to train for that goal. The more joy and fun you can bring to all of this healthy-living stuff, the better it's going to work.

2. In part 2, I explained why discipline, motivation, and willpower have totally failed you in the past, and hopefully convinced you that you need to ditch all the fad-diet/lifestyle attempts and focus on developing foundational habits. But not just any habits. If you want to get Healthy as Fuck, you want to cut right to the chase—to the keystone habits that require 20 percent of your effort and give 80 percent of the results: the 7 Habits of Highly Healthy Motherfuckers. To create these habits, you will establish a trigger, which will kick off the habit. Then, you will always get some kind of reward once you've completed the habit. If your habit doesn't feel inherently rewarding (yet), then you have to figure out a way to bribe yourself, because it's the reward that will automate the response between the trigger and the behavior. This is why it's so important to link joy to all of your new habits—in order to reinforce them. Do you see why I won't shut up about the happiness thing?

Now, here's the fun part—actually making this shit happen in real life. *Without quitting.* Because I'm guessing that you may have been here before. It probably occurred to you once or twice in your life that it might be a good idea to get some exercise. You probably even had a week or two of glory where you were Really Doing It This Time and you swore that you'd be at spin class each morning no matter what...until it's Wine Wednesday with the girls and you're all Britney-oops-I-did-it-again hitting the Snooze button, and then you get mad at yourself for being a Big, Fat Quitty McQuitterface.

Never again.

· CHAPTER 6 ·

THE LIFE-CHANGING, MAGICAL ART OF GETTING YOUR SHIT TOGETHER

LET IT BE KNOWN RIGHT NOW THAT NO ONE HAS EVER ACCUSED me of having an organized sock drawer. I have no idea what those washing instruction hieroglyphs mean on my clothes. I'm always caught by surprise when my kids have a holiday (and, let's face it, some Saturdays). My unpaid late fees are probably the real reason that Blockbuster Video went under. Maybe you are like me and your default self-organization skills leave something to be desired. Or maybe you are one of those people who in all seriousness asks for a label maker for your birthday and puffs up the pillows on the couch when no one is even coming over. Either way, you and I are gonna get our Martha Stewart on and experience the intense gratification—and subsequent results—of being totally on top of shit.

Here's why: your new habit loop isn't going to start executing itself just because you've decided it should; it's up to you to consciously create the conditions that will foster your new habits. Remember: If you want different results, you are going to have to do something different.

And often the biggest barrier to doing something different is simply a matter of environmental design. Here's what I mean.

I had a client who was having trouble exercising, which was kind of weird because she was hard-core and actually loved working out. But she couldn't get a regular habit off the ground, and she was really beating herself up about it. After I quizzed her for a bit, we figured out that the only time she could exercise consistently was first thing in the morning before her kids woke up. But then she didn't want to jump around because she'd wake up her kids. As soon as we were able to isolate this environmental barrier, we were able to solve it. I gave her a Silent but Deadly workout that involved no jumping but delivered the hard-core intensity that she loved. As soon as we solved this issue, exercise consistency was no longer a problem.

Another example: I was chastising myself for never being prepared with healthy food when I was on the move. I eat plant-based whole foods, and although I'm pretty creative, it can sometimes be a pain in the ass to find vegetables, like at a truck stop in northern Ontario, and I'd end up feeling like butt after scraping together a meal of corn nuts and stale pretzels. When I took a moment to think about why I never packed healthy lunches for myself, I realized it was because all my crappy containers leaked and I didn't want anything to spill in my bag. Once I had this blinding insight (no less earth-shattering than the Buddha's enlightenment under the bodhi tree), I was able to get my shit together and get some damn food containers that don't suck. Sometimes it's the little things that end up being the big things.

In this chapter, we are going to get super practical about how to:

- Deal with all the distractions and obstacles that have gotten in the way the other times you tried to do this habit.
- Remind yourself to execute the behavior after the trigger.
- Make it easier and more fun to actually do this shit.

This might sound like an ass load of work, but I invite you to get dorkily into it. Remember when you were little and you got all your new back-to-school supplies? The smug satisfaction of organizing all your new notebooks and binders? The anticipation you'd feel on filling a pencil case with the unused smelly eraser and freshly sharpened pencils? That sense that you were prepared for anything, armed and ready to unleash a year of academic brilliance that would leave the school no choice but to erect a plaque in your honor? That, my friend, is the Life-Changing, Magical Art of Getting Your Shit Together. Let's do this.

STEP #1: DECLUTTER

Once I was at a fitness conference and I went to a talk by a personal trainer who saved his little brother's life. His little brother was eleven years old and on the verge of morbid obesity. The personal trainer told us how he dropped everything and moved back home with his parents to try to save his brother. And week by week, his little brother started to lose weight. Finally, the trainer revealed a slide with an "after" picture of a beautiful, healthy boy smiling and flexing his baby muscles for the camera.

"Want to know what I did to help my brother lose all that weight?" he asked the room full of fitness professionals.

We leaned in, ready to take notes.

"I cleared all the junk out of the house."

THAT'S IT?! No big-deal-trainer workout? No nutritional strategy that solved everything? No Jedi mind tricks and psychological intervention? Nah, brah. Just get the fucking junk out of the house.

"But I don't eat junk," you say.

Of course not. Me neither. You are the kind of consumer who reads food labels, and books like this. But…there are some items that might have slipped your radar.

In The Kitchen

Your Trigger Foods

You know what I'm talking about. That food you love that is linked to all sorts of emotions and brain fuckery. You can probably even picture how much of it you have on hand right now. It might even be a healthy food. I know I can go to deep, sensual, and sometimes dark places with a tub of almond butter and a spoon. If it's a food you regularly eat in quantities that make you feel yucky, get rid of it. It's not forever. You can revisit having it around later, but while you are in the early stages of building your healthy habits, make it easy on yourself and get it the fuck out of the house. Oh, and stop pretending it's for the kids. If there was a moment in the past when it ended up in your mouth, there is a good chance it will end up there in the future. Just toss it or give it away.

And no, you don't get to have a big "last supper" where you get rid of it all by eating it. That is just inviting a binge-and-purge mentality and treating your body like a compost bin. That shit stops now. You are practicing loving your gorgeous, hot body exactly as it is, remember? And there is nothing self-loving about "cleaning up" by shoving excess food into your mouth. That goes for any eating you do when you aren't hungry, by the way. If you find yourself eating anything "so it doesn't go to waste," I need you to ask yourself: "If this food would otherwise be thrown away, why am I putting it in my body?"

That food is "a waste" simply by being more than what is needed. If you eat that food instead of throwing it in the garbage, it is still a waste, but in addition to that it is also doing harm to your body and making you feel like shit in the process. Just getting rid of the excess food will make you think twice before you buy or make too much food again.

(When I was on maternity leave, my mother's group would rotate hosting "playdates" where we would sit around and nurse and talk about our smashed pelvic floors and stuff. Someone would always bring treats—cupcakes and cookies that would get left like a grenade in the host's home after the horde moved on—until one brave mum ended it all, saying, "Get this stuff out of my house or I'll throw it into the garbage in front of you." I'm still grateful to her. None of us needed those treats, and she forced us to see that by bringing excessive food that no one needed we were all just contributing to waste.)

In addition to anything that is a head fuck for you personally, you also might want to chuck some stuff with shitty ingredients that can slip under the radar of even the most vigilant Healthy Motherfuckers.

Anything with "Sugar" in the Top Three Ingredients
I know I said that sugar isn't the devil, but remember you only get six teaspoons a day, so let's make those six teaspoons intentional choices instead of bullshit that's lurking in your cupboard. Remember that sugar also goes by any word that ends with *–ose.* You definitely want to chuck anything that has high fructose corn syrup, which has been linked to obesity, insulin resistance, increased belly fat, and heart disease. Sugar also has a bunch of code names you may not have been aware of, such as *maize syrup, glucose syrup, glucose/fructose, tapioca syrup, fruit fructose, HFCS (high fructose corn syrup),* and *fructose.*

Here's where you may find it lurking:

- Juice cocktails
- Any kind of soda (even tonic water)
- Breakfast cereal
- Yogurt
- Salad dressings

- Condiments (ketchup, marinades, barbecue or teriyaki sauce)
- Breads and baked goods
- Granola bars
- Nutrition or protein bars

Alcohol

I remember in my early working years feeling very grown up because I was accumulating a bit of a liquor cabinet. No retirement savings or anything, mind you, but my liquor cabinet was coming along nicely. Prior to this age of maturity, there was no such thing as a bottle of wine that happened to be sitting around the house, because all alcohol was consumed immediately upon purchase. (Who's got time to decant when there are more important things to do like drink the shit out of that wine?) Therefore, I considered it the height of sophistication when I started having casual bottles on hand to grab for drop-in guests or hostess gifts.

These are the bottles you might need to declutter. I don't know what level of maturity you are at when it comes to your liquor cabinet, but some of my clients need to get that shit out of the house. Bottles that get opened on a Wednesday night "YOLO moment" rarely make it to the weekend because, you know, "might as well finish the bottle." (YOLO = You Only Live Once. Just in case you spend less time listening to Canadian rap than I do. In which case you might want to add that to your fun list.) This was why one of my clients instituted a new rule that she and her husband would only consume alcohol at parties, bars, or restaurants. Not at home. Getting rid of the casual glasses of wine that were happening with dinner was a catalyst for better sleep, energy for workouts, and subsequent weight loss. (And let's face it—you don't need to keep those bottles around for hostess presents. Your hostess doesn't want another bottle of wine. She'll probably bring it back next time you host a party and it will become a hot potato the two of you throw back and forth. Bring a side salad so you can be sure to fill half your plate with vegetables, and save her from the pain of spiralizing beets to make a salad that looks fancy enough for company.)

Trans Fats

As I mentioned earlier, this shit is nasty and linked to heart disease, cancer, and diabetes. You'll find trans fats listed under code words like *shortening, partially hydrogenated, hydrogenated, monodiglycerides,* or *DATEM*. It's better to check the ingredients for those words; don't be fooled if you glance at the label and it says *Trans fat 0 g* because the FDA has allowed labels to list trans fats as *0 g* if the food contains less than 0.5 grams per serving. So the food manufacturer might make the serving size just tiny enough to get the "0 trans fat" label—even if it's not a realistic serving size. For example, a bag of microwave popcorn serves two and a half people. You try sharing one bag of microwave popcorn between two adults and a kid and see if anyone is happy.

Here's where you might find trans fats:

- Deep-fried foods (spring rolls, chicken nuggets, frozen hash browns, french fries)
- Frozen foods (quiche, burritos, pizza, pizza pockets, french fries, egg rolls, veggie or beef patties, anything with puff pastry or pie crusts, waffles, pancakes, breakfast sandwiches)
- Margarine and shortening
- Commercially packaged treats (doughnuts, danishes, cakes, pies, cookies, granola bars, puddings)
- Instant noodles
- Liquid coffee creamers
- Salty snacks (microwave popcorn, chips, crackers, even taco shells)

But listen—while you are going through your kitchen purge, try to avoid thinking that these are "bad" foods and you aren't "allowed" to have them anymore. When you put foods into "good" and "bad" categories, you are at risk for getting over-restrictive, and then having a rebellious backlash when you get the Fuckits, and then feeling all sorts of unnecessary guilt and shame. This kitchen cleanout isn't an exorcism of evil forces—you are creating some space for your new healthier habits, that's all.

And don't get mad at yourself for buying this stuff in the first place. The food industry doesn't make it easy for you to eat healthy, and not everyone has the luxury of scrutinizing every label that goes in their grocery cart. Especially if you've got kids. I know I'm not the only one who has ripped open a bag of crackers off the shelf to placate a toddler and buy myself time to find the damn almond milk before a full meltdown occurred. We all do the best we can, mama. Be kind to yourself and move on.

Speaking of being kind to yourself—here's the next purge you are going to make.

Your Closet

Give, throw, or pack away anything that makes you feel fat.

Yes, even those pants that you keep around because you hope to fit into them soon. I'm not saying you won't. If you start implementing the 7 Habits of Highly Healthy Motherfuckers, the zipper on those jeans is going to start cooperating in no time. But let's stop futurizing your life and remember that the point is to practice feeling hot and beautiful and confident and happy *now*. You want to start building those positive neural pathways associated with feeling good, to train your brain to access those feelings. If you are trying to access those feelings in a pair of pants that leave you out of breath and create big marks on your belly and give you a constant wedgie and pancake butt, you are making life harder than it needs to be. Remember that you can't "punish" yourself into getting hot and happy—that doesn't work. So ditch those pants that are being mean to you, and edit your closet down to those items that get you the closest to feeling hot, confident, sporty, and attractive RIGHT NOW.

You know what else feels good?

Digital Decluttering

We've done some pretty obvious decluttering of our physical environment, but the truth is that most of us spend a good chunk of our lives immersed in a digital environment. Now is a good time to think about this: Is there anything on my phone or on my computer that gets in the way of me executing my healthy habits?

For example, my client Danielle was having a tough time getting to her 6:00 a.m. boot-camp class because as soon as her alarm went off, she would reach over and start scrolling through her social media in bed. Before she knew it, she had missed class. Once Danielle took the social media apps off her phone, she got up, got dressed, and was out the door in time for her class. If that's too extreme for you, I've got some other ideas coming up to prevent social media from taking over your life. But also have a think about:

- Are there news apps that you have a habit of checking right before bed that stress you out?
- Do you need to clear some videos from your phone so you have room for your new running app?
- Do you get annoying notifications when you are trying to meditate?
- Do you follow any Instagram accounts that make you feel shitty about yourself?
- Do you want to get extreme and cancel your Netflix or cable for a month so you aren't tempted to watch *Mad Men* again instead of going the fuck to sleep?
- Is it time to delete Candy Crush and start crushing some workouts instead?

If you want to create some hard boundaries around general media consumption in order to free up some time and head space, one idea is to install the Freedom app, which will block certain sites for you. Danielle, for instance, could have used Freedom to block Facebook until after her class was over. I have other clients who have used Freedom to initiate a hard end to their workday by disabling their email client after 5:00 p.m., which forced them to chill.

Whatever your digital situation is, it's worth taking a look at your phone and computer and scanning for anything that:

- Stresses you out
- Wastes time without really making you happier
- Triggers you to eat or drink alcohol
- Prevents you from sleeping
- Distracts you when you know you should be meditating or food prepping or exercising

Now, don't get me wrong—I'm not saying that your digital world is a menace to your healthy habits. But instead of being technology's bitch, you want to use it to get so hot and healthy that cartoon birds and squirrels flutter around like you are a Disney princess.

Step #1 of the Magical Art of Getting Your Shit Together is decluttering, and we've freed up some extra space in your digital and physical world. Now we need to add some reminders to your environment, so you actually remember to do your new healthy habits.

STEP #2: CREATE REMINDERS TO DO YOUR
NEW HEALTHY HABIT

Remember that "poke" feature on early Facebook? What if instead of getting poked for no fucking reason by someone you barely remember meeting, you instead poked yourself to do your fucking habit like you are supposed to?

This is where technology can be your BFF. There are some amazing habit apps that you might want to consider downloading, now that you've done your digital declutter. For a full list with links, go to www .fitfeelsgood.com/book, but here's a preview:

- Rabbit (iOS) will send you notifications at prechosen intervals to take a break, drink some water, etc.
- Persistence (iOS) allows you to see statistical analysis of your habit patterns.
- Stikk (iOS and Android) has the option to put money on the line if you don't stick with your habit.

But that's not the only way your phone can help kick-start your habits. Even without downloading an app, you can use the native Apple Sleep function to set your intended sleep schedule, and it will play a lullaby when it's time to settle down for the night. You can ask Siri to remind you that it's time to go to the gym when you leave work.

Basically, if your trigger is time- or location-based, your phone can call you out and remind you to do it.

If you are more of an analog kind of Healthy Motherfucker, you can also use old-school physical reminders, like:

- A Post-it Note on your computer reminding you to meditate before you dig into your email
- Obstructing your front door with your gym bag each morning
- Posting your meal plan on your fridge

I have one client who sleeps in her gym clothes so she is reminded as soon as she wakes up that she'd better get to the gym. I have another that keeps all her hair products at the gym, so she's forced to go if she doesn't want to go to work looking like a Chia Pet.

It's showtime, Synergy! (*Jem and the Holograms* reference? No?) Time for you to write down at least three ways that you are going to remind your ass to execute your habit after your trigger.

But the real question is: How are you going to design your environment to make your new habits fun and easy? Because that's when the act of Getting Your Shit Together really IS life-changing.

STEP #3: DESIGN YOUR ENVIRONMENT TO MAKE YOUR HABITS MORE FUN AND EASY

In my early days as an actor, I worked for a film production company run by a dominatrix. And much of her workforce (not me, let's be clear) were actually her lovers who would work for free in exchange for occasional humiliation and degradation. Needless to say, it was a fascinating work environment. And not because of the weird sex stuff (that happened after hours and wasn't evident to me during work hours), but because my boss was a model of someone who took complete control of her company—and her life. She accepted absolutely ZERO shit. And by "shit" I mean the normal life stuff that you and I would just think we have to suck up. To her, the only acceptable outcome was that everything happened in a way that was "fun and easy." There was no complaining tolerated because it was inconceivable that anyone would grind through a task that was mind numbing. She set a standard for maximum enjoyment of life and she deliberately designed her environment to meet those expectations. It was either fun or it wasn't happening. You might be rolling your eyes at the idea of refusing to ever vacuum your house again (or maybe you are wondering how you can get some love slaves to do it for you) but for my dominatrix boss, the difference between something being mundane and being "fun and easy" was largely a matter of outlook. That's why production meetings would start with the primary question "How could we get this job done in a way that would be fun and easy?"

By insisting that the best way to get every job done was to make it fun and easy, my boss created a work environment where *jobs actually got done*. And they got done well. By people who were having fun and not complaining. Because of that, we got unbelievable results in every respect. We won awards that we shouldn't have qualified for. We got grants that made no sense. We got media accolades and connected to powerful people. Fun and easy. It always worked. This is where the life-changing magic part comes in.

In this section, I am inviting you to take control and dominate your life, and demand that your new healthy habits be fun and easy. Enough with tedious to-do lists of virtuous tasks that feel like a yoke around your neck. No longer will moving your glorious body feel like a chore. No longer will eating healthy feel like chewing cardboard and sadness.

> **Take control and dominate your life, and demand that your new healthy habits be fun and easy.**

Here are some ideas, listed by habit, of ways that you can make doing this shit EASIER and have more fun doing it.

Fill Half of Every Plate with Vegetables

- Buy a sauce or condiment that you really love. I will eat a napkin if you put spicy pesto on it, so bring on the brussels sprouts.
- Get a plate with a visual of what proportion should be veggies.
- Cross off each day of the calendar that you hit your seven servings a day.
- Investigate weird-ass vegetables like jicama and fennel to break out of a carrot-and-celery rut.
- Buy your veggies already processed: washed and julienned or spiralized or whatever. Yes, it costs more. But if you eat the vegetables, it's worth it.

Go the Fuck to Sleep

- Buy a good fiction novel to help you unwind screen-free.

- Get an old-school alarm clock to keep your phone away from your bed.

- Check YouTube for guided sleep meditations or bedtime stories. There's one about a balloon that I do with my kids that will put me in a coma.

- Invest in some fancy bedsheets and put some lavender under your pillow. It really doesn't take much to feel like you are treating yourself to an indulgent mini-spa.

Back Away from the Booze

- I've had a lot of clients substitute their alcohol rituals with sparkling water like LaCroix or with yummy teas.

- If you like to drink a glass of wine with your partner in the evenings while you watch TV, could you substitute the wine for taking turns giving each other a shoulder rub? You'd get a similar feeling of physical relaxation and bonus points for building your relationship with potential sexy times.

- Sobriety Counter is an app that gamifies your nondrinking, showing you how much money you've saved and challenging you to a memory game that will help you ride out the scientifically proven three minutes of craving a drink.

Chill Your Ass Out (and Meditate)

- Download one of the excellent meditation apps like Calm or Insight Timer, and let someone walk you through your meditation so you can just relax and ride the chill.

- Treat yourself to a beautiful journal.

- Tell Siri to automatically go into Do Not Disturb mode for twenty minutes while you meditate at 8:00 a.m. each morning.

- If you are someone who wants quantifiable evidence that this meditation shit is actually doing something, you could invest in a brainwave-sensing headband. You can even get competitive with your friends about who is the most chill if you are that type. (And if you are, seriously, it's meditation time.)

Eat It All, but Eat Way Less of It

- Consider getting one of those bento-box-style lunch boxes, which will take care of your portions, and you can be all Harajuku-girl adorable.

- Download the app Eat Slowly to eat more mindfully.

- Prepackage your food into serving sizes. For example, don't have a big Costco-sized bag of trail mix sitting around. Divide that shit up into smaller portions. (I had a friend once confide in me that he had a fantasy that he was buried alive in a bag of Costco trail mix and had to eat his way out. I wish I could say I can't relate. That's why I need to make portion control easier on myself and divide into the little portions.)

- Use smaller plates. Most of us have been wired to clean the plate. Don't try to fight it—just eat off a smaller plate and watch your intake go down automatically.

Prep and Plan Ahead

- Sharpen your knives and dig out that food processor you bought at a garage sale.
- Blast music you haven't heard since high school while you prep.
- Make a Pampered Chef Party host extremely happy by investing in the Deluxe package so you are ready to package and store your healthy food.
- If you have grocery delivery available in your area, consider scheduling an automatic delivery on Sundays (or whenever you want to do your prep).

Exercise Consistently

- Sign up for a local class. That way you don't have to think about what to do—and you might not believe me, but it really is more fun to exercise with other people.
- Remember what was fun for you as a kid and figure out how to do it more. I love dancing, and I go to an event called No Lights, No Lycra every week. A bunch of us get together in a dark room and dance. That's it.
- Make sure your shoes fit, your pants don't bunch up, and your bra does its damn job.

- Get obsessed with a podcast that you treat yourself to while you get moving.
- Download some sick new music on your phone.
- Check out your local used marketplace for any gadgets you think might help you get moving. Almost everyone has an Ab Roller gathering dust and broken dreams in their basement, and they are happy to unload it. Workout programs, dumbbells, and healthy cookbooks are the stuff that fuels the garage-sale economy. I got my Fitbit on Craigslist for $40, and it's been motivating me to move for two years now.

These are the three essential steps to the Life-Changing, Magical Art of Getting Your Shit Together:

1. Declutter
2. Create Reminders to Do Your New Healthy Habit
3. Design Your Environment to Make Your Habits More Fun and Easy

If you take these steps, you will be well on your way to making sure you start executing your habit after your trigger, allowing the reward, and thus your brain will start hardwiring your awesome new habits to make you thin, powerful, and gorgeous.

But before we leave this chapter, I want to emphasize that for most of us, the biggest factor in the Life-Changing, Magical Art of Getting Your

Shit Together is creating and protecting your personal time. I told that story about my dominatrix boss for a reason. Not only did she insist on tasks being fun and easy, but she *took charge of her own life*. She would never whine about not having enough time because she knows that we all have twenty-four hours in the day, and how we spend those hours is up to no one but us. Too often I hear my clients play a victim role in their own damn lives and try to squeeze their healthy habits into the space that's left over after they've met everyone else's needs. Let me tell you something right now: everyone else will keep demanding from you if you let them. It is your job to create hard boundaries about when you are available. You have to put yourself first. That's not selfish. That's responsible.

And I know you are reading that and thinking *but-but-but the kids, the job, the house.* I'm not saying you have to let all of that go up in flames in the pursuit of health and hotness. What I am saying is that if you have a couple of bucks to spend on your wellness, it's very possible that buying back your *time* will be the way to spend them. As I've mentioned, it's very possible that your best health-and-wellness investment would not be another piece of fitness equipment, but a housekeeper and a babysitter.

At the time of writing, these services cost about $10 to $30 an hour in my market. If you have a limited budget for healthy living, skip the boutique spin studio at $40 a class and buy yourself an hour or two where the kids are happily entertained and the house is clean. Use the time to meditate, go for a jog with a friend, or prep some healthy meals while singing at the top of your lungs.

Doesn't that sound more fun and easy?

· CHAPTER 7 ·

THE POWER OF YOUR PEEPS

WHEN I WAS IN SEVENTH GRADE, MY FAVORITE T-SHIRT WAS white with neon-orange writing in a funky '80s font that said *Normal Is Boring*. I wore it with acid-wash jeans and two different colored shoes and thought I was really sticking it to The Man. In high school, I briefly (but with maximum public fanfare) smoked a pipe. In my twenties, I was cast in a role for a play that I thought was misogynistic, so I not only grew out my leg hair but *mascara'd* it for performances. School sports? No thank you. If you need me, I'll be wearing too much eyeliner and smoking behind the school. Team spirit? I'd rather die.

Yes, I was a total pain in the ass.

The reason I'm admitting to being an adolescent Rebel Without a Fucking Point is to illustrate that I am not someone who is naturally a "joiner." But even though my teenage self is wincing as I admit this,

I am now the queen of camaraderie; of organizing team challenges, of getting a group together to run the race in oh-so-kooky matching tutus, of rallying the troops and yelling, "Come on, guys, we can dooo it!"

It's massively dorky. And it Totally. Fucking. Works. I mean, you can keep smoking a pipe and rolling your eyes at group activities if you want to, but I'd rather be healthy, hot, and happy. And for that, you need your peeps.

Here's why: Normal isn't just boring. Normal is:

- Obese or overweight (60 percent of North Americans)
- Stressed (77 percent of Americans)
- In debt (49 percent of Americans)
- Underslept (35.3 percent of Americans)
- Binge drinking at least once a month (26 percent of Americans)
- Not moving nearly enough to be healthy (80 percent of Americans)

And I don't want any part of that. At the risk of repeating adolescent patterns, I will say that "normal" can go fuck itself. As old-school motivational speaker Jim Rohn once said, "If you are not willing to risk the unusual, you will have to settle for the ordinary."

And in our society, it's pretty damn unusual to be fit. It's not normal to be the kind of person who moves their body, eats healthy food, declines the second drink, sleeps, meditates, and preps their healthy food in advance.

But there's another important part of what Jim said that you might have missed: it's a risk to be unusual. Humans much prefer to adapt behavior to conform to societal norms. Sensing social disapproval can actually trigger our brain's danger systems, which makes sense from an evolutionary perspective. In prehistoric times, being part of a tribe was the only way to bring home the mammoth. Our great-great-great-grandmothers who didn't conform to social norms in medieval Europe were burned as witches. As recently as my childhood, little boys who wore pink faced merciless schoolyard bullying (until *Miami Vice* came along and made everything okay).

The human tendency to conform is well-documented, but probably the most famous example is the 1950s study by Solomon Asch in which volunteers were told they were taking a vision test to see which lines were the same length.

LINE TEST

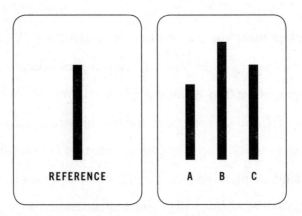

A replication of the cards used during the experiment. The card on the left is for reference; the one on the right shows comparison lines.

When asked alone, they chose the right line. But when asked in a room full of other "participants" who chose the wrong line, the subject would choose the same line as the others, even though it was clearly the wrong answer.

Even my teen rebel wannabe self got totally busted in a conformity demonstration. I once arrived at my drama class to find that chairs had been placed around the room, and one of my classmates was standing on one. I followed suit, as did every other student who arrived. Soon, all the students were standing on chairs, and the teacher walked among us silently for a while as we awaited further instructions. Were we being trees in a forest? Practicing "trusting" the chair? Really, anything is possible in Drama 101. Finally, the teacher said, "Why the fuck are you guys all standing on chairs? I didn't tell you to do that!" And we all protested that everyone else had been standing on chairs. She smiled and suggested that we might want to start thinking for ourselves.

Which is easier said than done. We all have this idea that we are independent thinkers. But the ironic fact is that one of the greatest predictors of nonconformist behavior is having a backup of allies and social support. Nonconformist behavior is most strongly associated with the presence of allies. Valuing rugged individualism is a huge part of the American psyche and cultural identity, but the myth of the lone cowboy is pretty much bullshit. Look for the successful revolutionist and you'll also find a group of supporters. To be honest, there's no way I would have been ballsy enough to mascara my leg hair before going onstage if I hadn't had a couple of friends backstage who thought it was hilarious.

My whole point here is that if you are going to succeed in swimming against the current of society by getting Healthy as Fuck, you are going to need your tribe. You need people to join your rebellion. You need to find a new normal to which you can conform without succumbing to the societal default of fat, sick, tired, and stressed. You need the Hogwarts that will be your refuge in a world full of Muggles.

Not only is it helpful when you are trying to build a new habit (your peers will remind you, they will make it more fun), but if you don't want to be a Big, Fat Quitty McQuitterface, you will definitely want to get some peeps on your side because, consciously or unconsciously, you will crave their approval and that will help reinforce the habit loop.

Which is why my online transformation program includes meal plans, workouts, "go-get-'em-tiger" emails, and...a Facebook group. Every now and then someone will say, "I don't need the Facebook group. Just give me the recipes and the workouts and I got this." I get that—I really do. No one needs to spend more time on social media, and who cares about a bunch of strangers and what they ate that day, right?

Except that a Facebook group will create a new cultural norm to follow. One study found that online weight-loss communities can play a prominent role in weight-loss success. Participants in the study found the group important for encouragement (87.6 percent), information and practical tips (58.5 percent), as well as a sense of shared experience (42.5 percent). People think what they need is a magic formula of workouts and recipes, but the real magic formula is surrounding yourself with people who are also living Healthy as Fuck. People who will be cheering you on. People who believe that you can actually do it (even when you have those moments that you don't think you can do it). People who set a social standard for doing it, so you feel like you not only want to do the habit, you *have* to.

> People think what they need is a magic formula of workouts and recipes, but the real magic formula is surrounding yourself with people who are also living Healthy as Fuck.

So please: join a team, get a running buddy, invite someone over so you can do Meal Prep Power Hour together, find a fitness class that you love, join an online program with community support. By the way—if this thought makes you queasy because you are afraid you will be the worst one in the class, or you will be slower than your running buddy, that's totally understandable. I'm going to tell you how to get over that in chapter 9. But for now, just know that if you are going to get Healthy as Fuck, you need to find people who are already doing your healthy habit and who are genuinely supportive. You need the people who will be happy for you, rather than trying to make you feel all weird about changing...which brings me to your friends and family.

Friends and family might not be your best social support system when you are getting Healthy as Fuck. In fact, they might be kind of assholes about it. A Stanford University study showed that 75 percent of women "rarely or never" got support from friends or family in their weight-loss efforts. Another study found that one fifth of people admitted to trying to sabotage friends' weight-loss efforts. When asked why, respondents said their healthy friend got "too boring," or their friend's healthy living made them feel bad about themselves, or they were straight up jealous of the results their friend was getting.

Remember the conversation between Michelle and Jennifer earlier in this book? It went like this:

> **Jen:** "I'm on a diet! I want to lose ten pounds so I can look like a smokin'-hot MILF at my son's bar mitzvah next month!"
>
> **Michelle:** "What? That's *ridiculous*! You don't need to go on a diet! You're perfectly fine the way you are!"

As I pointed out, although it might seem like Michelle is just being a stand-up, I-love-you-just-the-way-you-are friend, she is also (a) stating her opinion about Jen's body, which is totally irrelevant, and (b) squashing Jen's ambition.

It's also possible that Michelle's (probably totally subconscious) motives for squashing Jen's ambition have less to do with wanting Jen to love herself and more to do with Michelle needing to love herself.

If Jen loses ten pounds and looks like a smokin'-hot MILF at the bar mitzvah, then what does that do to Michelle's relative hotness status? If Jen suddenly starts exercising, how does that make Michelle feel about being totally out of shape? If Jen starts drinking Perrier on girl's night, does that shine a harsh light on Michelle's wine-stained teeth and slurred speech?

Here are a few ideas for dealing with friends, family, and colleagues who are (again, probably unconsciously) trying to sabotage your results.

1. MAKE SURE THEY DON'T FEEL JUDGED.

People are funny—you tell them you want to get healthy and they immediately make it about them. Be clear that your choices are just about you, and they won't be so reactive. Consider this scenario: You go to a restaurant, and for the first time, you ask the waiter which options are vegan. Your friend asks what's up.

> **Option #1:** "I just think that eating meat is perpetuating an inter-species genocide that will horrify generations to come, and anyone participating in it is destined to burn in the fiery pits of hell."

Or

> **Option #2:** "Yeah, I just find that my digestive system feels better when I don't eat animal products."

Here's a social pro tip that etiquette expert Emily Post never mentioned: When wanting to avoid a conversation about your diet, allude to "digestive issues." It will shut the conversation down ASAP because (a) no one wants to picture you pooping, and (b) no one feels morally judged when you allude to suffering from wicked dairy farts. You having a fucked-up stomach lining doesn't mean that I have to reconsider my Krispy Kreme habit. Everyone is happy. To be honest, the old "digestive upset" strategy is why I think the faux–celiac disease diet works so well.

2. DON'T BECOME BORING.

If you think that following your healthy habits means that you have to stay at home and avoid restaurants and parties and social situations:

> you will definitely not stick to any of your new habits because your life will suck, and
>
> you will get pressured by all your friends and family to give it up—and rightfully so, because it probably isn't making you happy.

I know that when you are first trying to navigate your new healthy habits, it can seem easier to just stay home and skip the movies rather than have to face Han Solo's death in Episode VII without a tub of buttered popcorn on your lap. I mean, I'm getting triggered right now just thinking about what a dick Kylo Ren is, and some buttery popcorn would probably make me feel better (temporarily). But there comes a time in all our lives when we have to adult the fuck up and practice living as healthy people who can enjoy a movie without trans fats and about 300,000 unnecessary calories. The kind of person who can go to a party and have two drinks instead of twelve. Warning: If you do pause the enjoyment of your life and your relationships, that's an indication that you are seeing this as a temporary diet, rather than your new awesome way of life.

Don't be boring, and people can't accuse you of being boring. (And if your friends' idea of "boring" means "not shit-faced drunk," then you might want to go friend shopping.)

3. DISGUISE IT.

There are people who are going to feel hella triggered by you not eating a slice of birthday cake at the office party or whatever, and that is their shit. But it's annoying to deal with and usually these casual acquaintances are not worthy of getting the riveting details about your "digestive issues" (see option 1), so you might just want to disguise your healthy habit. Stuff like this will usually work:

- Take the cake but don't eat it.
- Say you are full but ask if you can take the delicious cake home with you (where you are free to pitch it or give it to someone else who will enjoy it).
- Say that you have a big dinner planned and want to save some room.
- Go to the bar and order a soda water with lime, which looks enough like a cocktail that no one asks questions.

4. DISTRACT.

The thing to remember is that when people are upset about your healthy choices, it's never about you—it's about them. So distract them by turning the subject back to them. Examples:

> "No thanks, I don't need a piece of cake, but I want to hear about how the big presentation went today! I heard you killed it!"

Or

> "Nah, I'm going to stay sober tonight, but that means I can drive and that will save us a buttload of cab fare! What time do you want me to swing by to pick you up?"

You'd be surprised how supportive friends can be of your healthy habits when it makes life more convenient for them.

5. TRY TO CONVERT OR ASK FOR SUPPORT.

I would save this for only your dearest people, like your immediate family and close friends. You might find some resistance, but it's pretty critical to your success. Besides, it will make your new habits so much more fun and easy if your boo is on board. When I used to do one-on-one training, I would always ask people how their spouses felt about their new healthy habits. Because if the spouse isn't on board, I know that my client is on a countdown to relapse. There's only so much you can do to fight against a spouse who doesn't want to spend extra money on organic food, who wants to keep your nightly glass of wine ritual, who resents you being unavailable during your long runs. Here's what you need to do:

1. Explain to them in advance what you are trying to accomplish.
2. Tell them why it's important to you.
3. Reassure them that you aren't being all crazy.
4. Ask for their help, and be specific.
5. Acknowledge that it might be a sacrifice for them.
6. Thank them.

Here's a sample script a mom could use to talk to her family:

"Hey, guys, can I talk to you about something important? I want to lose some weight and get in awesome shape. I know you love me exactly the way I am, and I'm so grateful that I have your unconditional love, but this is something that I want for *me*. I want to feel like my old self, I want to feel more energy, and I want to feel more confident. Most of all, I just want to prove to myself that I can do it. I'm actually really excited. And don't worry, I'm not going to stop eating or do anything dangerous. In fact, I'm using a new habits-based approach that feels sustainable for the very first time. I wanted to tell you guys about this because I know I'm going to need your help if I'm going to achieve my goal. It will make me feel so good when I do. Will you help me? (Get agreement.) Here's what would be really helpful: Kids, do you think you could make your own lunches in the morning so I can make mine? That way we can all eat healthy food during the day. Honey, do you think you could commit to being home on Monday, Wednesday, and Friday evenings so I can go to my new salsa-dancing class? And would you guys be okay if we tried some new healthy recipes? We might miss some of our old favorites, and I can't promise you are going to love each new recipe, but we never know if we don't try, right? And we can still order in pizza as a special treat every Friday. Is that a deal? And Honey, I'm going to hold off on the wine until the weekend. Would you help me out by not offering me wine at the end of a hard day? And maybe encourage me to actually go to my salsa class, even if I say I don't feel like it? Tell me that I'll feel better if I go even if I say I'm too tired? Thanks, guys. I know that sometimes it can be hard when things change, but I really think these changes are going to make me much happier, so thank you so much for helping me make them happen. I love you!"

Or, if that speech is not your style, you could copy my client Sandi's genius speech to her family:

"Okay, listen up. This month is all about ME. And I expect your support on this. I've been driving you guys around to soccer practice and cooking your favorite meals for ten years. It's my turn. No one is allowed to talk to me until my workout is done in the morning. And we are going to be eating my food. With lots of vegetables. And no complaints. If you don't like it, there's a lasagna in the freezer. *And* you can reheat."

Mic. Drop.

My teen-rebel self wants to come out of retirement just to start a new Riot Grrrrl band and make Sandi's speech the lyrics to an aggro anthem of feminine empowerment. I think it would be a big hit.

But there was one crucial difference between these two speeches. Sandi's was awesome, but she forgot an important element when asking for social support. Did you catch it? She forgot to ask for help in calling out her bullshit.

· CHAPTER 8 ·

BREAK UP WITH YOUR BULLSHIT

MY FRIEND MINDY HAD A SHOE PROBLEM THAT WAS GETTING out of control. It's not easy to spend more on Reeboks than rent, but Mindy was giving it a solid go. Until one day she announced she had achieved Peak Shoe. Her closet was now complete, and Zappos was just gonna have to find a way to stay in business without her. And then she showed up in another pair of new shoes. I asked about them, and she said, "I know I said I wouldn't buy any more shoes, but these were an end-of-season sale. It's just smart to buy them now. This way I won't buy later."

Further footwear transgressions were explained in different ways:

"I actually kind of bought these for my boyfriend. He always
wants to go for hikes, and I never had the right shoes to go
with him. He's going to be so happy!"

"Well, these don't count because I had to buy them for work. I
    don't even like them that much."
"These are my reward-for-not-buying-shoes shoes."

In each case, Mindy was completely convinced that she had an
ironclad defense for breaking her stated intention not to buy shoes.

But let's face it—this is Bullshit. Bullshit is the stories we all tell
ourselves so we can feel okay about not sticking with our intentions.
You might hear this kind of thing referred to as loopholes. Gretchen
Rubin very eloquently discusses loopholes in her book *Better Than
Before*. But I think "bullshit" is the only way to properly describe
the mental shenanigans people use to sabotage their habits—and
themselves. Here's how the Bullshit will show up for me.

My alarm clock will go off for my early morning workout and—I'm
not gonna lie—sometimes my first conscious thought is, *Fuck. Me. I have
to go do my workout now. I seriously don't feel like it today*. And that's
when the Bullshit Marching Band starts parading through my head.

Baton girl in front: "You don't have to work out today! You worked
really hard yesterday and you deserve a day off!"

The drum section: "It's just one workout. One workout doesn't
matter when you've been so good. It's raining out. Fuck it."

The horns are jubilant: "You can skip one day! Jeez! Live a little!
Enjoy your life in this moment!"

Finally, the tuba will fart some flaccid promise: "Go back to sleep
now and maybe you will work out later today?"

That last effort of my brain is so laughable that not even my laziest self can believe that I might actually do a workout later on in the day when in forty-two years there is zero historic precedent for an afternoon workout ever happening.

But man, is it ever tempting, delicious bullshit. This Bullshit is the brain equivalent of getting a witty text from an ex who wants to come over.

Well, hello there.

> **The reason that the Bullshit is so seductive is because it lets you relax into the familiar—and postpones the pain and discomfort of moving on with your damn life.**

You know it's such a bad idea. But in the moment, it can seem so right. Best damn idea anyone has ever had.

The reason that the Bullshit is so seductive is because it (like the text from the ex) lets you relax into the familiar—and postpones the pain and discomfort of moving on with your damn life. We've all learned that giving in to the temptations of your ex coming over is a horrible idea—we know it will just keep us stuck in old patterns. Same goes for the temptations of giving in to the Bullshit You Use to Squirm Out of Your Habit.

We want to give in because our Bullshit allows us to stay in our comfort zone without feeling too bad about it. Which is exactly why this Bullshit is the mental excrement in which fledgling good habits go to fester and die. This is the thought trash that is the corrosive acid to your Healthy as Fuck lifestyle.

It's time to truly break up with your Bullshit.

In order to defend your habits (and your self-respect), you must implement my patented Three-Step Process to Break Up with Your Bullshit:

1. Recognize your Bullshit. See that it is Bullshit.
2. Deliver a kind but firm breakup speech.
3. Do your damn habit anyway.

Recognizing your Bullshit is the first hurdle.

At this point of maintaining my healthy habits, I can lie awake in bed watching that whole Bullshit parade tromp through my head and not fall for its witty banter and flirtations. I know I'm just lying in bed wasting energy, wildly trying to think up excuses, instead of sleeping *or* exercising. I know I just have to get the fuck up and get the workout done, and that not wanting to is just part of the deal sometimes. That the real muscle I need to strengthen is the "get the fuck up even when you don't feel like it" muscle. (I don't always want to exfoliate my skin, pay my phone bill, and go to other people's kids' birthday parties either, but sometimes you've just got to adult the fuck up.)

Now do you want to know the best way to unmask your Bullshit and reveal it for the stinking saboteur that it has always been? Meditation.

I know that 99 percent of the fair readers of this book read the word *meditate*, rolled their eyes, and gave the meditation habit a hard pass, thinking that it's not gonna help you get back into your premium denim. But meditation is where you train your brain to observe your thoughts. Most of us go around believing that we *are* our thoughts and that every piece of mental puke we conjure up is true. In a lot of cases, this keeps you believing old thought patterns that are seriously unhelpful: *I just have a low metabolism. Exercise just isn't my thing.*

The only way to free yourself from these thoughts is to find a way to observe them with a bit of detachment: *Huh. There I go thinking that thought again. That's interesting.* That detached observation of our thoughts is what we practice during meditation. And don't worry—it's not like you have to be fucking Yoda or anything in order to recognize the Bullshit You Use to Get Out of Your Habits. By the end of this chapter, your favorite Bullshit should be embarrassingly clear.

Once you recognize your favorite Bullshit, you can move to step two of my Anti-Bullshit Artillery: the Breakup Speech. This is where you start to compose the exact words you are going to use next time this Bullshit shows up and wants to hang out—and hold

The real muscle I need to strengthen is the "get the fuck up even when you don't feel like it" muscle.

you back. Be gentle but absolutely firm. I've given you some ideas, but your Bullshit is going to need to hear it directly from you in order to get the message that it's truly over.

And then you will proceed to the third and most crucial step of Breaking Up with Your Bullshit: Do Your Damn Habit Anyway. I know that you aren't always going to feel like it—and I don't demand that you are always perfect. I do, however, demand that you are honest with yourself. So ditch the Bullshit and just admit you don't fucking feel like it. In the next chapter, I'll tell you how to make these habits so easy-peasy-lemon-squeezy that you won't even be tempted to squirm out of them.

But for now, let's meet the eager contestants that are trying to seduce you and help you squirm out of your habit. I'd like to introduce you to: your Bullshit.

THE DIET-STARTS-TOMORROW BULLSHIT

Every now and then one of my clients will ask if they can "pause" my healthy-habits program because they are going on vacation. Or things are crazy at work. Or something unexpected has come up.

And the answer is no.

Diets get paused. Habits are *who you are.*

Case in point: My lovely client Holly signed up for my program during a year that turned out to be the hardest of her life. Her dad was sick. Holly spent the year traveling across the country and staying overnight in hospitals when she wasn't looking after her young son. If Holly was on a diet, that diet would have been over fast. But her healthy habits sustained her. The exercise and healthy food helped keep her sane, healthy, and strong enough to handle the shit storm and tragedy that life was throwing at her.

If things are bad enough that you start thinking *I can't deal with my healthy habits now*, it's probably when you need your healthy habits the most.

On the other hand, if things are so *awesome* that you start thinking *The diet starts tomorrow (because today I'm on vacation, it's my birthday)*, then you might want to ask yourself why you wouldn't want to feel good on your vacation, or on your birthday. (Just a friendly reminder: that's what you are ultimately working on here—making yourself feel good. Happiness. Remember?)

If you want to give yourself the "treat" of putting your habits off until tomorrow, it's a sign that you are seeing your habit as a punishing pain in the ass. It's a good clue that you need to strengthen the reward part of the habit loop.

Here are other versions of this Bullshit that I hear a lot:

"This weekend is a write-off. I'll start fresh on Monday."

"I'll order dessert now and just do a hard workout tomorrow."

"I'm going to enjoy the holidays, and I'll deal with it in January."

Can you recognize this sweet seduction? Tempting, right? The idea that our future selves will be better behaved is a great way to excuse a current transgression.

But it is mental garbage and also physiologically based on a false premise. You can't "work off" food by doing extra exercise later (as discussed already), nor can you neutralize a binge with a cleanse. That's just not the way the body works. Do you get strong arms by doing one thousand push-ups in one day? No. That's how you get injured. Your body hates that shit. You get strong by doing ten push-ups for one hundred days. Remember—your body will respond to consistency over extremes. Does that mean you are totally fucked if you do have a wild weekend? No. It just means that you return to your regularly scheduled program of

> The idea that our future selves will be better behaved is a great way to excuse a current transgression.

healthy awesomeness as soon as you decide that the party is over. And you don't need to wait until Monday to have the freedom to start fresh.

If you've ever seen a bumper sticker on a hippie van, you know that the only moment you really have any power over is the one that's happening right *now*.

Here are some breakup speech ideas for when your brain is trying to convince you that the Diet Starts Tomorrow:

"Even though I'm on vacation, I'm still going to moderate my alcohol because I want to feel good and energized to enjoy my vacation to the max."

"Even though I'm so slammed at work right now, I'm going to take the time to meditate, because this is when I need that sense of inner calm most."

"I don't have to finish this whole meal just because I ordered it. I can put down this fork and ask for the rest of this meal to go. I'll be so happy that I didn't overeat and will enjoy these leftovers later."

"I got wasted last night, and I'm too hungover for my workout today. But instead of lying around and eating hangover food today and then 'starting on Monday,' I could drink a big glass of water and go for an easy walk in dark sunglasses."

"I'm starting to feel the toll of too many holiday parties, but I don't have to wait until the New Year to feel better. I can make a salad right now and see if my family wants to go for a walk."

"I started a new episode of *Game of Thrones* even though I know I should go to bed and get my seven hours of sleep. That doesn't mean that I can't turn off the TV at any moment and reverse the decision. The rest of the episode can wait."

"I'm halfway through my vacation, and I've totally relaxed my habits. But that doesn't mean I have to wait until I get home to get back on track. It starts with filling my plate with vegetables at the next meal."

Every moment is a chance to start fresh. Not just Mondays. Not just January. Even halfway through a binge, you always have the power to bring some awareness to the moment and make a new choice. Claim that power.

THE MARTYR BULLSHIT

Sometimes the tempting Bullshit that bubbles up is that keeping to our habits would actually make us a bit selfish. It would be an act of kindness and graciousness to forego our habits just this once.

I'll be honest—my brain loves this particular Bullshit. I crush out on it so hard because it's so appealing to believe the only reason I would ever bail on my healthy habits is because I'm pretty much Mother Teresa. It sounds like this:

> "I should probably try all these hors d'oeuvres because the hostess went to so much trouble to make them."
>
> "I should skip my fitness class tonight and stay home with my kids. They want to play with me."
>
> "It would make my friend feel uncomfortable if I didn't have a glass of wine with her."
>
> "If I take time for myself to do meal prep on Sundays, then my husband will have to take the kids to swimming lessons, and he really likes to sleep in. That wouldn't be fair to him."

It's so much fun to think of ourselves as altruistic in our choices, but this is Bullshit because we are actually *using* other people to defend our own actions. It's not cool. When you play the altruism card, you become like the aging mother who is always guilt-tripping her kids and saying how much she gave up for them. What a shitty thing to do to your kids. If you get caught up in this Martyr Bullshit, it's time to cut it out now.

Here are some breakup speeches to try:

> "The best thing I can do for my kids is to be happy and energized

with them today, and healthy so they don't have to take care of me in the future. It is my motherly duty to ditch them and go take care of myself."

"If my friend is uncomfortable with me not drinking, that's because she is questioning her own drinking. When I provide a casual and nonjudgmental model of someone having fun and not drinking, I'm doing her a favor without being preachy."

"My hostess wants me to enjoy myself. If I overeat, I will feel uncomfortable and not have as much fun at her event. There are plenty of people here to freak out over her hors d'oeuvres."

So enough with the Martyr Bullshit. Put the oxygen mask on yourself by following your healthy habits, and then you will be healthy enough to Mother Teresa all you want.

THE AHA-MOMENT BULLSHIT

I know this might come as a bit of a shocker given all the Cool Kid Street Cred I established in the previous chapter with my different-colored shoes and everything...but I am a total self-improvement junkie. I was secretly listening to Tony Robbins's *Personal Power* cassette tapes when most of my friends were listening to Nine Inch Nails. I love diagnosing people's Love Language two minutes after I've met them. I do Power Poses in bathroom stalls before meetings. You call them grocery lists—I call it Food Goal Setting.

Which is why I am particularly susceptible to the Aha-Moment

Bullshit. It's when you have a sudden burst of personal growth that allows you to squirm out of your habit. It sounds like this:

"I know I said I wasn't going to eat desserts, but I believe in living in the moment and this cake looks delicious. After all—you only live once!"

"I know I said I was going to exercise consistently, but actually, I've decided that I love myself the way I am and I don't need to make myself work out if I don't feel like it."

When you hear yourself using Aha Moments to get out of your healthy habit, it's a good time to review the difference between pleasure and happiness. As I mentioned at the end of part 1, pleasure comes from external circumstances (dessert, sleeping in) and is fleeting. Happiness comes from within, is stable despite our circumstances, and comes from being in alignment with our core values and identity. Happiness comes when you are making real progress toward goals that are meaningful, and there's usually a bit of grit required to do so. Pleasure is the temporary feeling of relief when you relax into the familiar. It's cuddling on the couch with your ex instead of moving through the discomfort of being lonely. It feels good in the moment, but deep inside, you know it's not right.

It is very hard to be truly happy when you are not following through on your stated intentions. That's how you know that these Aha Moments are total Bullshit.

Here are some break up speeches:

"Yes, I only live once. So, I want to spend my one life feeling
energized, healthy, and awesome. Eating that dessert wouldn't
make me feel that way."

"Yes, I love myself exactly as I am. And I believe I can do anything
I set my mind to. It's because I love myself that I am totally
committed to pushing through challenges and achieving my
greatest potential."

"My highest and most awesome self would just do my damn habit
right now. You know it. I know it. That's who I want to be. So
let's do this."

THE VICTIM BULLSHIT

This is where you pretend that aw shucks, you wish you *could*
exercise—if only your gosh-darn kids would leave you alone long
enough to do it!

Other examples would be:

"My boss ordered a bottle of wine for the table. I had to drink some!"

"My knees hurt when I exercise, so I can't."

"I wish I could meditate, but I'm just not wired for it."

"I can't focus on eating healthy and finding vegetables right
now—work is just too crazy."

"I'm too old to start exercising now."

This is an especially smelly brand of Bullshit because it is so disempowering and, frankly, makes you sound like a wuss for not taking control over your damn life. And if you believe that you are a wuss who doesn't take control of her life, then there's a whole bunch of shit you aren't gonna do—and I'm not just talking about burpees.

Here are some breakup speeches for the tempting Bullshit that you believe is beyond your control:

> "If there are athletes in the Special Olympics who manage to be in incredible shape with no legs at all, I can probably manage to figure out a workout that accommodates my grumpy knees."
>
> "I noticed that Sam from the HR Department didn't drink the wine, and she didn't get fired. Maybe no one would care if I didn't drink."
>
> "Meditation is hard for everyone. I'm no exception. In fact, that probably means I could benefit from it even more."
>
> "Yup, it would have been great if I started to exercise twenty years ago. But the second-best time to start would be right now. Studies show that the best thing for older adults is to get active."
>
> "Who do I know who manages to have both a family and a consistent exercise habit? Mary is evidence that a mortal human can get both of those things done."

When sniffing out the Victim Bullshit, you want to pay special attention to your language. For example, I don't let my clients use phrases like "I fell off the wagon this weekend" or "I went off the rails during my vacation." Both of those suggest that you have no power over your life, which is why the Victim Bullshit is the *most dangerous Bullshit of all*. I'd much prefer to hear "I decided to get maximum value for my all-inclusive vacation and stay drunk for seven days."

I'm not saying that's a good decision, but it's a hell of a lot more empowering than being all "Whoopsie daisy! I couldn't help myself!" about your freaking life.

The funniest thing about the Victim Bullshit is that if you rewind the tape, you will often see that you inadvertently created your victim circumstances and set yourself up in a situation where you were destined to fail. Stuff like:

"I'll totally do my meditation after I check my work email."
"I'll order the fries, but I'll just eat one or two."
"I'll let my ex come over, but just so we can be good friends."

Bitch, please.

We all know how this is gonna turn out. It's as predictable as watching a horror movie where a group of teenagers decide to rent a cabin in the woods and the wild girl decides to go skinny-dipping. Carnage is inevitable.

Here's how you are going to break up with this Bullshit. When you hear yourself coming up with some silly-ass plan like—

"Let's just go to Disney World with three kids, and I'm sure we'll all be motivated to find the healthy and affordable food that I'm sure is readily available."

Or

"Oh look! My favorite ice cream is on sale at the store! It would be smart to stock up now and just keep it in the freezer for special occasions."

—then I want you to think to yourself:

"Am I setting myself up for success here? Or am I being the girl who goes skinny-dipping at the haunted cabin?"

Don't be that girl, dude. That girl put herself in a situation where she was destined to be a victim. Instead, be the girl who unexpectedly knows kung fu and escapes the cabin to live another day. Or, you know, at least the girl who orders the damn salad instead of thinking she is gonna eat two fries and then sit there in front of a plate of delicious fries with zero interest in the rest. Be the girl who shows up for the road trip with healthy snacks. Be the girl who brings her sneakers on vacation. The girl who makes sure she has childcare coverage for her exercise classes. The girl who doesn't open her work email until the meditation is done rather than pretending she's a victim of work getting crazy and that's why she can't meditate.

THE GOOD-GIRL BULLSHIT

Wouldn't it be nice if someone patted you on the head and told you that you were such a good girl and that you deserve a treat?

Hell yes it would. About damn time someone realized all the shit I do around here and how diligent I've been with my healthy habits. You are damn right I deserve a treat. I've really been very good—it won't even matter if I break my habit and have a treat just this once.

This is the Good-Girl Bullshit. These tempting mental flirtations might include:

"I've been so good with my habits—I deserve a weekend off."

"I just worked out really hard this morning, so it's okay if I have a treat."

"I've been so good, so it won't make a difference if I skip my workout this one time."

"I've been so good that one little cookie won't hurt."

To most of us, the feeling of deserving-a-treat/Good-Girl Bullshit is the most familiar. It's easy to get sucked into this Bullshit because it's partly true; you probably are being "good" all the freaking time—fulfilling duties and expectations and running around getting things done.

Remember that human beings will always be motivated to seek pleasure. And if you are always working, and looking after people, and attending social events that aren't fun for you, and cleaning the house, and paying bills, and generally not experiencing any pleasure… you will eventually snap and demand a treat for yourself.

I tell my clients to imagine that some part of them is a little kid that a parent is dragging through a bunch of boring errands in a crowded shopping mall on a tight deadline. The kid is overwhelmed, tired, hungry, and grumpy—and the parent never lets them stop and look at any toys or just goof around. The kid is just supposed to behave and "be good." Eventually that kid will protest that she has been good enough and will have a full-on fucking meltdown if she doesn't get to do something fun or get soothed with a treat.

Now obviously the ideal solution here is to not put a kid in that situation and not let the kid get to the stage where she is overwhelmed and underslept and tired and hungry. But we often don't do that kind of preventive self-care. We expect too much from our little-kid selves, which is why I suggested in the previous chapter that maybe the best thing you could do for your health is figure out how to make your life just a little easier and fun.

The best way to break up with the Good-Girl Bullshit is to work on making your habits feel less like dutiful chores and more pleasurable. It's time to beef up the reward part of your habit loop. When you go around thinking that you "deserve a day off," you are telling yourself that your habit is something hard and horrible. Instead, we want to be training our brains to associate pleasure with our habits.

Breaking up with the Good-Girl Bullshit might sound like this:

"Yeah, I've been so good with my habits, so I don't want to break the streak! I deserve to see the results that come from consistency."

"I worked out really hard this morning, so I should fuel my body
with something nutritious. It's going to taste so good, and I'll
feel awesome."

"I've been so good with my habits, I totally do deserve a reward.
What would a Healthy Motherfucker such as myself do for a
kick-ass reward?"

It's also easy to convince yourself that you are so good that one little time doesn't matter. It's true: One cookie won't make you fat. And one workout won't turn you into Halle Berry (which is a serious bummer).

The fact is that every single time counts, which is why it is so important to be vigilant about our Bullshit in the first place.

Remember how the habit loop works? You have a trigger, then you do your habit, and then you get some kind of reward. Every time the habit loop happens, it gets wired more deeply in your brain. Do it often enough and eventually it happens automatically, and then you get to spend your time learning the guitar or running for mayor or making seashell necklaces or whatever the fuck you want to do with your life that isn't worrying about how to get Healthy as Fuck. So that's awesome.

But.

Every time you have the trigger and you DON'T act out your habit, you are making the loop weaker. You also make it less likely to become automatic, which means it will be a little harder to do the next time.

Which is why you need to:

1. Recognize your Bullshit.
2. Deliver a kind but firm breakup speech.
3. Do your damn habit anyway.

I know that you might have been reading this with your heart sinking as I slayed some of your favorite Bullshit patterns. Maybe you were thinking, *Really? Like, I have to fill my plate with vegetables every day forever and ever? And if I skip it on my birthday, I'm fucked forever?*

Nope—you aren't fucked forever. It's about doing your best absolutely every single day without letting your Bullshit suck you back into a relationship (with old patterns) that you've outgrown. And trust me, you have outgrown this Bullshit. If you can recognize it, then already you are developing an immunity to its charms and you are ready to move on.

And no, that doesn't mean you have to be absolutely perfect with your habits every day. In fact, if you try to be perfect, *that's* when you are totally fucked. If you demand absolute perfection from yourself, you will go crawling back to your Bullshit for relief and feel like a failure.

In the next chapter, I'm going to teach you how you can be delightfully imperfect with your healthy habits and still keep them happening on autopilot. You are going to love this.

· CHAPTER 9 ·

IF YOU CAN'T DO SOMETHING RIGHT, DO IT TOTALLY HALF-ASS

EVERY NOW AND THEN I WILL HAVE A CLIENT WHO INFORMS ME with pride that they completed my transformation program perfectly. Every workout crushed. Every green smoothie gulped. And I secretly think *Oh shit* because I know they are heading for a crash. Worse, they probably have an identity invested in being someone who does things perfectly. And let me be the first one to tell you that there is no fucking way you are going to execute all your new healthy habits perfectly. Why?

- Because you are a guest at someone's house.
- Because you are sick.
- Because drinking Bailey's at 8:00 a.m. on Christmas morning with your dad is awesome.

- Because holy shit, that's not sparkling wine; it's real Champagne.
- Because your mom made you that marshmallow sweet potato casserole thing because she thinks it's your favorite.
- Because sometimes you Just Won't Want To.

Moments like these will bring you to an inevitable fork in the road. And thinking you have to do this *perfectly* is the Highway to the Danger Zone.

But before I get into the giddy delights of Doing Things Totally Half-Ass, let me admit that I can relate if you are someone who likes to do things right. I used to walk around saying macho shit like "I'm an all-or-nothing kind of person" and "If I can't do it right, then I don't do it at all."

I was actually pretty proud of this all-or-nothing identity until my first day of acting school. Remember that school I told you about where we spent a month of higher education trying to tiptoe out of a room silently? Yeah, that was actually a really hard school to get into. We flew from all over the world to London, England, to audition for a few select spots. So on the first day, the rest of the chosen ones and I were sizing one another up when this guy sits next to me and, with a big smile and a lovely Birmingham accent, says, "I hope I'm the shittiest one in the class. That way I'll learn so much!"

I was totally gobsmacked. I realized I would *die* if I were the shittiest one in the class. I would absolutely die. I would go home and never speak of this whole acting thing again. When he positioned being a shit actor as an opportunity for improvement, it was the first time I was able to see my big wall of an ego that insisted I had to do it right or not do it at all.

(By the way, if you found my recommendation to join a group totally barf-inducing, there's a good chance it might be because you don't want to be the shittiest one in the group. Which is so understandable. But if you can leave your ego aside long enough to shrug off that very real possibility, you are setting yourself up for a massive leap forward. Because when you have the balls to put yourself in situations where you suck, when you have the courage to hang out with people who are so much better than you, it forces you to level up.)

Before my Birmingham friend bitch-slapped me with some self-awareness, I (like many people) unconsciously avoided any situation in which I was destined to suck. It's absolutely the reason I skipped gym class when I was a kid—I am definitely not naturally athletic. To this day, if you threw a Frisbee at me, my first instinct would be to charge you with assault.

It's a natural human tendency to avoid stuff you aren't good at. It's cool. We all have egos to protect. But there is no growth in being perfect at something. And the need to be perfect has prevented a lot of people from allowing themselves to get Healthy as Fuck.

I don't even want you to *try* to be perfect at all your new habits. There will come a moment when you can't deal with your new habit, I can guarantee it right now. I hereby give you loving permission to Do It Totally Half-Ass. The best part is that this half-assery will actually lead to better results! Let that sink in for a second, my Type A friend: When you give yourself permission to occasionally do things totally half-ass, you will actually get better results than if you demand constant perfection.

It looks like this:

Can't deal with your 5K run today? Just go for a walk around the block and then give yourself all kinds of mental high fives for your athleticism.

Can't handle another plate of vegetables? Add an extra topping of green peppers to your pizza, some cocktail onions to your martini, and pat yourself on the back for being a winner.

Not enough time to squeeze in an hour of meal prep? Pull something healthy from the freezer so it's thawed for later and give yourself massive props for setting yourself up for success when you come home hangry.

Habit experts like Charles Duhigg, author of *The Power of Habit*, call these "small wins." Small wins are going to rock your world and free you from the all-or nothing weight-loss roller coaster once and for all. Here's why.

SMALL WINS REINFORCE THE HABIT LOOP

Remember that our goal here is to get your healthy habits on autopilot. You've got better shit to think about than remembering to execute your new habits—and the world needs your brain power focused on bigger things than eating enough vegetables. In time your habits will automatically happen when you consistently execute the behavior after the trigger and then allow the reward. Every time you follow the pattern, you are taking a step toward making that behavior as instinctive and automatic as your teeth-brushing loop, or the loop that makes you check your email constantly.

The key is to not break your healthy habit loop—even when you seriously can't be fucked to do it. The good news is that the loop can still be reinforced if you execute a smaller version of your habit. For example, if your habit loop normally looks like this:

Trigger: It's 6:00 a.m.
Behavior: Go for a forty-minute run and listen to the podcast *Serial*.
Reward: Knowing what happens in *Serial* and exercise-induced endorphins.

On days when you have a cold, the loop might look like this:

Trigger: It's 6:00 a.m.
Behavior: Go for a walk around the block while listening to *Serial*.
Reward: A *Serial* hit and exercise-induced endorphins.

And it still totally counts.

This habit loop will still be strengthened—even if it's a smaller version of the habit—as long as you continue to allow the reward. So, it's important to give yourself all kinds of gold stars, even when you half-ass it. How fun is that?! It's like being back in Little League soccer (the peak of my personal sports career). Everyone gets a trophy as long as they show up. Fist pump! Here's why small wins work so well:

SMALL WINS REINFORCE YOUR HEALTHY MOTHERFUCKER IDENTITY

This is critical. According to my boyfriend Tony Robbins, "The strongest force in the human personality is the need to stay consistent with how we define ourselves." If you have phrases you use to define yourself, like "I'm just a neat freak!" or "I'm a perfectionist," you will move mountains to maintain that identity. So if you go around saying shit like "I'm not a morning person" or "I'm just lazy," guess what? You will never get up and work out—even if you think you really want to. This was a lesson I learned when I was trying to quit smoking. I wanted to quit. I intended to quit. The only problem was that I strongly identified with being a Smoker. I had created this (very stupid) teenage worldview that *Smokers = cool, creative, counter-culture, independent thinkers* and *Nonsmokers = lame, boring, conservative losers.* Which made it very hard to quit, despite my conscious mind (and wheezing lungs) recognizing that it was definitely time to give up the ciggies. I still considered myself at heart a Smoker (who was just not smoking right *now*), which set me up for certain relapse. Only once I revised my identity to officially be a Nonsmoker (and revised my idea of what that meant) was I able to make a lasting change in my behavior.

Now, let's again take the previous example:

Trigger: It's 6:00 a.m.

Behavior: Go for a forty-minute run and listen to the podcast *Serial*.

Reward: Knowing what happens in *Serial* and exercise-induced endorphins.

But imagine that instead of executing a small win (going for a walk around the block), you roll over and go back to sleep.

This will weaken the habit loop as mentioned above, but even worse, it also weakens your identity as Someone Who Does This Shit. You will start to lose trust in yourself.

Every time you roll over, you are fueling self-doubt and giving power to the Bullshit identity that might be keeping you stuck.

Every time you get up and do the smallest of small wins, you are solidifying your new identity as someone who does what they say they will do. You strengthen your belief in yourself and cast a vote for yourself as the Healthy Motherfucker you are meant to be.

SMALL WINS LEVERAGE MOMENTUM— AND YOUR EGO WORKS FOR YOU!

Let's continue with the above scenario. The alarm goes off at 6:00 a.m. You are supposed to go for your habitual 5K run, and you seriously don't fucking feel like it. You watch your brain come up with all kinds of Bullshit about why you don't really have to do it. You know it's all Bullshit, but that doesn't change the fact that you are grumpy, and you just don't want to. So, you promise yourself today will be a small-win day. You get up with the intention of doing ten jumping jacks in your living room and then going the fuck back to bed. But once you are up and moving you figure that you might as well go for a walk. And then once you are outside and walking, your ego pushes you to try a little jog. And before you know it, you've fulfilled your habit to a much greater extent than you intended when you were negotiating with yourself in bed. And you're probably way less grumpy.

So don't be surprised if your pitiful, grumpy-ass attempt at a small win leads to a snowball effect of you being kind of fucking awesome.

SMALL WINS MAKE YOUR HABITS BULLSHIT-PROOF

The beauty of small wins is that they are kryptonite to your Bullshit. Even the most creative, enticingly sexy Bullshit won't give you a good reason to squirm out of your habit if your habit is so tiny that it's ridiculous to apply a bunch of Bullshit to get out of it.

For example, let's say I'm absolutely convinced that I do not have time to meditate for twenty minutes.

My brain: *No way. Too busy. My disengagement from my work for the next twenty minutes could result in a catastrophic global economic meltdown. Nope, not even ten minutes. If I close my eyes for ten minutes, I will fall behind on my work, and I don't know how I'm ever going to catch up at this point. I'm sorry, no, not even five minutes to spare. I'm already late for my next thing. Could I take a deep breath? Umm...yeah, I guess. Okay there, I did it. I meditated. Yay me! I guess the world didn't collapse after all...*

(By the way, the above mental script is only a minor exaggeration of some classic Victim Bullshit.)

Do you see how Doing Things Totally Half-Ass can surprisingly be a total game changer when it comes to actually sticking with your habits? You will reinforce your habit loops and your identity as a Healthy Motherfucker. You will also put your powerful ego to work for you and get more done than you otherwise would have as well as neutralize the Bullshit that have made you quit in the past.

Not convinced? Listen, I've worked with a lot of high achiever Type A people (they tend to be the ones hiring top trainers, obvi) and they are generally very much all-or-nothing, go-hard-or-go-home types. Consequently, they are also often stuck in the weight-loss roller coaster pattern of going balls-out on the latest trend diet and then crashing spectacularly when shit gets real. Here's an example of how I've used small wins with them.

I used to train my client Debra at her house at 9:30 a.m. on Tuesdays. And usually we'd go run up hills and do strength training and all kinds of fun, hard-core stuff. But every now and then I'd show up and she'd open the door and say "SHIT. I'm so sorry, I should have called you. There is NO WAY I'm working out today. I didn't sleep a wink last night, I'm so stressed out."

I'm sure she was desperate to get rid of me. But I knew that if I went away, then she'd be breaking the habit loop we had created for Debra:

Trigger: It's Tuesday at 9:30 a.m.

Behavior: Exercise with Oonagh.

Reward: Sense of well-being and social affirmation from Oonagh.

So instead of taking the fucking hint and leaving, I'd invite myself in and empathize about the rough night. Not as a strategy or anything—it sucks to be stressed out and have insomnia. She was absolutely right in thinking that it's not a great day to do hill runs and strength training. I would commend her for listening to her body. But that doesn't mean we can't execute a small win. Instead of skipping the workout entirely, I suggested we do some stretching, deep breathing, and talk about stress-management strategies. In doing so, we were reinforcing Debra's habit loop:

Trigger: It's Tuesday at 9:30 a.m.

Behavior: Stretching with Oonagh.

Reward: Sense of well-being and social affirmation from Oonagh.

We also:

- Strengthened Debra's identity as someone who makes time for self-care.
- Weakened the idea/Bullshit that stress and fatigue mean she can't take care of herself.
- Reinforced the idea that stress and fatigue mean she has to take *extra* care of herself.

Now do you see how awesome and totally essential small wins are when it comes to getting Healthy as Fuck? And how it can be the essential missing strategy for you wonderful all-or-nothing people?

Start thinking of the...

teeniest

tiniest

shittiest

stupidest

what's-the-fucking-point

...version of your habit.

Keep getting smaller and smaller until it would be absolutely ridiculous to believe the Bullshit that you can't do that teeny-tiny version of your habit. This way you are armed and ready with some appropriate half-ass effort when the necessity arises.

To save you the brain power, I've got some half-ass inspiration for you:

"I don't have time to make a week's worth of healthy meals in advance!"

Could you chop up some veggies to have on hand for snacking?

"I can't handle another salad, and I want something yummy."

Could you throw a few leaves of spinach into a blueberry smoothie?

"I slept through my boot-camp class."

Could you do the Scientific Seven-Minute Workout at home?

(Listed here: www.fitfeelsgood.com/book)

"There's no way I can get seven hours of sleep each night."

How about at least going to the bedroom fifteen minutes earlier

than usual?

"I can't survive on appropriate portions. I'm still hungry!"

Could you wait five minutes before getting a second helping?

"I need my glass of wine in the evenings. It's my treat."

Could you try a half serving for one night and see how that feels?

"I can't handle meditation."

Can you handle taking some deep breaths and counting to ten?

Now here's the fun part: you get to reward yourself just as enthu-siastically as you would if you did the full version of your habit. In fact, you *must* in order for the habit loop to be fulfilled. So, instead of thinking of that walk around the block as a failure to go for a run, think of it as a success in getting off the couch. Then, think of how it might affect the quality of your life if you allowed the small wins to feel like real wins and celebrated them every day.

Remember that it's not about being perfect, but just a little bit better. And by the way—you do have to get better. You can't just go putting three leaves of spinach in your blueberry smoothie for the next three years and think you are fulfilling your veggie requirements. These delightfully half-ass efforts are your insurance against plunging into the Fuckits because they disarm the all-or-nothing mentality. Small wins allow a minimal acceptable version of your habit to serve as a placeholder until you are ready to get back to the business of your regularly scheduled awesomeness. As you progress on your journey as a Healthy Motherfucker, you will find you need your small wins less often, and you will naturally raise your bar on what you consider a minimally acceptable version of your habit.

Instead of thinking of that walk around the block as a failure to go for a run, think of it as a success in getting off the couch.

But for now, just remember that every little bit counts toward that compound-interest chart. Anything is better than nothing. Every tiny positive action is a vote for the kind of person you want to be. And again, changing your *identity* is what is going to make this Healthy as Fuck approach different from every other time you have tried a diet or "eating healthy."

That's why you should be doing the mental equivalent of football touchdown dances every time you:

- Choose the salad instead of the fries.
- Wind down with a book in bed instead of starting another episode on Netflix.

- Remember to pack healthy snacks.
- Get up and stretch after sitting in front of your computer too long.
- Have one cookie instead of three.

If you acknowledged each of these small wins with a mental Academy Award acceptance speech, wouldn't that make you feel kind of awesome?

And, just a reminder, it's all about feeling good and loving yourself NOW.

CHAPTER 10

HOW TO FIGHT THE FUCKITS

AND NOW, LOVELY READER, IT'S TIME FOR YOU AND ME TO HAVE The Talk. Have a seat.

I wanted to discuss something that may be a little uncomfortable, but it's perfectly natural and there's no reason you should feel embarrassed. You have come very far in your journey as a Healthy Motherfucker. And I am so proud of you. Around this time, you might start to notice some changes in your body. And that's a good thing! It means you are blossoming into the strong and healthy woman you were meant to become. But sometimes, when we go through changes, we can also have some very strong emotions. These emotions are called the Fuckits. Have you ever found yourself thinking thoughts like:

"I know I said I was going to eat healthy, but fuck it, fast food is just easier."

"I know I said I wasn't going to drink during the week, but fuck it, I've had a hard day."

"This healthy-habit stuff is a pain in the ass. Fuck it. Pass the brie."

Yes, I thought so. It's totally normal. And even though the Fuckits can feel really yucky sometimes, they are actually an important part of growing up.

The Fuckits are like the puberty before you hit full maturity as a Healthy Motherfucker. This is the inevitable stage when you want to give up on your new healthy habits. The Fuckits make you moody and grumpy. You might feel like you don't even know who you are anymore. You will feel rebellious, defiant, petulant—and *totally pissy*. The Fuckits aren't a flattering stage. But (like puberty), they are a necessary part of you blooming into your full potential. The challenge is making it through to the other side of the Fuckits and crossing the threshold into a new phase of maturity and wisdom, where your healthy habits are on autopilot and having abdominal muscles is no longer just an urban legend.

It's a phase that most people never reach. Those kids are still riding the diet roller coaster, and for them, the Fuckits mark the crash of their latest diet effort, the moment they declare the diet (or, much more tragically, themselves) a failure.

To show you where the Fuckits fit into the life cycle of a Healthy Motherfucker, here is my perversion of the Transtheoretical Model of Behavior Change (possibly the most studied framework of healthy behavior change in psychology).

In this model, there are six stages we go through when changing our behavior or habits:

1. **Precontemplation:** Our future Healthy Motherfucker is sitting on the couch playing video games and eating pizza pockets. It really doesn't occur to her to want to get healthier. She has never Googled a sugar-free recipe and thinks Zumba is an African language.

2. **Contemplation:** Okay, she's still sitting on the couch, but she's starting to feel kind of guilty about it. Every now and then she might announce that she is going to get in shape, but it's still all talk at this stage.

3. **Preparation:** Now we are getting somewhere. She's splashed out on some new Nikes, she's reading books like this one, she's got some kale sitting in her fridge that she might actually eat, and she even called the gym for pricing options. She's basically gassing up the tank and revving the engine at the starting line.

4. **Action:** And she's off! Our girl is doing shit for real. This is

a moment for self-celebration, for developing structures to support the new habits and gathering lots of high fives from peeps who support her.

5. **Maintenance:** At this stage she's been at it consistently for a while now. She's developing self-sufficiency, solid habit loops, and feels successful. On the other hand, the initial thrill has worn off and she sometimes feels bored or complacent. Or sometimes she just gets compliance fatigue. If she doesn't remember to reinforce her new healthy habits, it can lead to the next stage.

6. **Relapse:** Otherwise known as the Fuckits. Because that's when she says, "Fuck it. I'm sick of this shit. Pass me the game controller, and can you heat me up a pizza pocket? I don't want to get up."

Catastrophe? Hardly. Here's why you shouldn't beat yourself up if you have a case of the Fuckits.

THIS SHIT IS TOTALLY NORMAL

I'm not saying aim for the Fuckits or anything, but nothing in life progresses in a linear fashion, so there's no point in freaking out when the Fuckits show up. Your goal is to pull yourself out of the slump quickly and with minimal drama. I'll tell you how to do that in a paragraph or two, but first let me repeat: nothing in life trends upward in a perfectly straight line. No one's career is just one promotion after

DOW JONES

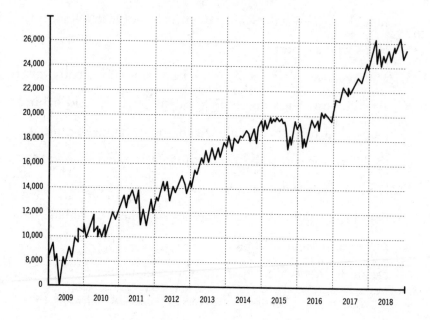

another. No one's relationship is just peachier every day. And certainly no one's health and fitness is one "personal best" day after another. Even when things look like a steady upward climb from a distance, there are always the peaks and valleys within that general trajectory. For example, the chart above shows the Dow Jones over the past ten years. It's generally going up, but you can see that there is a jagged pattern within that upward climb.

And if you zoom in to just the latter half of the last year, you will see the jagged pattern within the jagged pattern, meaning that we will have good months and bad months. Zoom in a bit more and you'll see good days and bad days. Good moments and bad moments.

So you don't want to sweat those downward drops too much.

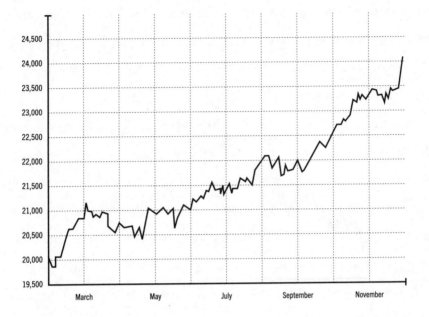

ZOOMED DOW JONES

Instead, you want to pull back the camera and ask yourself whether your progress is generally trending up or down. Here's how you can make sure: If your progress is trending upward, then the highs will be increasingly higher and the lows *will also be higher*. If you're trending down, your lows will be lower and your *highs will also be lower*.

Here's what an upward trend might look like with our healthy habits:

- Highs are higher: I just ran for twenty minutes straight for the first time ever!
- Lows are higher: I went on a bender last night but drank vodka and soda instead of my usual white Russian cocktails.

See? The high was a bit higher—she not only went running, but she also pushed a little bit harder than ever before. The low was also a little bit higher. She doesn't have to be perfect and never go out drinking. Her overall health is trending upward because she did it just a little bit healthier than last time.

Even if your Fuckit spiraled from a few vodka and sodas to a bender that would make a frat boy blush, remember that creating habits isn't about perfection. Habit-building is the slow process of re-establishing what your norm is—or what "home" is to you. It's not that you never go on a trip (or a one-night bender); it's that you always come back home (to your healthy lifestyle, your new identity).

I heard a story once about a martial arts master who could stand on one leg forever. His students marveled that he never lost his balance. The master corrected them and said, "I'm always losing my balance; I just find it very quickly now."

And that's really the deal. As you master your new habits, you will find that the Fuckit phases will get shorter and less frequent, and you'll go less deep into them. That's partly because you are building habit automation, but also because you will have done your research. This brings us to another reason why you shouldn't sweat the Fuckits too much.

YOUR FUCKIT RELAPSE CAN BE REFRAMED AS RESEARCH

Once you've been consistent in doing your healthy habits for a while, being a Healthy Motherfucker will be your new normal. This is awesome, obviously, but it can also lead to thoughts such as *I feel fit and awesome. I don't need to keep doing all these healthy habits anymore.* It's like the person who goes off their medication as soon as they start to feel better, not realizing it's *because* of the medication that they feel well. These thoughts might tempt you to conduct highly scientific experiments like the following:

Observation: I sure feel like a fine specimen of humanity these days!

Question: Do I really need to keep doing all this healthy-living shit?

Hypothesis: Maybe I can now resume my old habits with minimal consequences. I predict that if I relax all my healthy habits, I will be happier and feel freer.

Experiment: I will spend this holiday season eating and drinking whatever I feel like and exercising only when it's convenient and I'm in the mood.

One month and five hundred puff pastry hors d'oeuvres later

Conclusion: Hypothesis not supported. Although the initial thrill of relaxing my habits was fun, I quickly found that my energy and confidence were impacted, and the result was less happiness.

If you need to do some research, then do some research. But fer fuck's sake, don't deny yourself the lesson you learn from your research. Gain the knowledge and get on with your damn life. Spare yourself the energetic resources of conducting the same experiment over and over again, mmmkay? Even if you do need to—*ahem*—confirm the results of your initial findings by testing again ("Maybe I should try partying my way through vacation and see if it's a different outcome than the holidays!"), reframing your visits to Fuckitland as a deliberate experiment is so much more empowering than saying something like, "I fell off the rails."

Because guess what? Sometimes your hypothesis will be supported! Maybe you *will* be happier if you loosen the reins a bit.

Which brings us back to the beginning of this book—where you get to *choose*. Remember back in chapter 1 when I insisted that you get to choose the body you want? The way out of the Fuckits is to start back at the beginning and repeat the process I've outlined for you in this book. Starting with...

STEP #1. EXERCISE YOUR RIGHT TO CHOOSE.

Now that you've conducted your experiment, you have great data to use to help you choose where you want to be on your effort-to-results ratio chart. Remember that each individual has their own effort-to-results chart, and you get to pick the right spot for you on that continuum. You either:

Choose the effort you want to give and make your peace with the consequent results.

Or

Decide on the results you want and accept the effort required to achieve your goal.

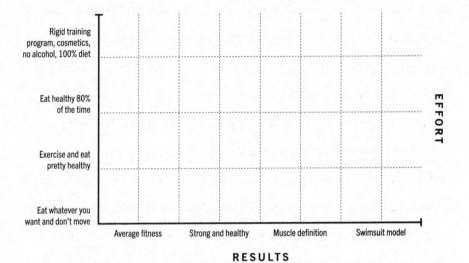

Now that you have more information about what level of effort feels sustainable and what results are most important to you, you can be more intentional in choosing the perfect spot on that chart for you. You are better equipped to determine the right balance between the effort you're willing to put in and the results that will make you happy.

In yoga there is a saying that each pose should have a mixture of Sthira (strength or structure) and Sukha (softness or sweetness). Your Healthy as Fuck lifestyle should aim to strike a similar balance. Most people will quickly find they are unhappy without structure, even if they think they want to "be free." In fitness, that structure looks like regular exercise and healthy eating habits, regardless of whether you feel like it in the moment. Having total "freedom" to follow what you feel like doing in the moment—hitting the snooze button, eating whatever looks delicious—is confusing immediate pleasure with the pursuit of deeper happiness. Deeper happiness comes from the personal growth afforded by accomplishing hard goals. And accomplishing hard goals requires some structure.

On the other hand, most of us will rebel if we are caged within structures that are too strict. Again—it's about balance. Pleasure, sweetness, and freedom are important. If you never eat anything sweet, never miss a grueling workout, and never stay up late to party with a good friend, it's probably only a matter of time before you snap. If you find that you are getting the Fuckits too often, maybe you are demanding too much Sthira/structure and not enjoying enough Sukha/sweetness. Maybe you need to choose a different spot on your effort-to-results chart.

I've already told you that I chose a spot that results in me having a belly—even though I'm a leader in the fitness industry. Stereotypically, my position means that I should be inspiring you with pictures of my ripped abs, shiny hair, and perfect meals on Instagram. But I'm afraid you'll have to do without that kind of inspiration because I've experimented with habits that resulted in a very lean body, and although I loved the look, I found the structures too hard to maintain and not worth it—for me. I've also experimented with total "freedom," which resulted in a much bigger belly and lower energy, and it made me unhappy, unhealthy, and uncomfortable in my skin.

And so I've chosen a place on my personal effort-to-results chart that includes a bit of a belly. It also includes some killer biceps I love, burpees I do even when I don't feel like it, the occasional beer I enjoy immensely with a summer sunset, and brussels sprouts I eat automatically just to fill half my plate with vegetables. This is the perfect Sthira and Sukha for me. Whether the outcome inspires people is not something I have control over. My responsibility is to choose consciously and then get to work on loving both the effort and the results.

If you've had a bout of the Fuckits, it's a great time to review and recommit to where you want to be on your effort-to-results chart. If you choose deliberately and radiate the happiness that comes from that choice, I will find you inspiring as fuck, and I'll totally follow you on Instagram. ;-)

Now, what if you've chosen exactly where you want to be on your effort-to-results chart but are struggling with executing your habits consistently? In that case, move on to step 2!

STEP #2. DO YOU HAVE THE *F*s?

Now that you've chosen the perfect spot on your effort-to-results chart, you might want to check your pockets to make sure you have sufficient Fucks to maintain the effort you've chosen.

Remember that if you want to see different results in your body, you are going to have to do something different with your habits. This will require extra Fucks when you are first establishing your habits and they are not yet happening automatically.

Revisit the pleasure and pain exercise that you totally skipped back in chapter 3. What are the real consequences if you don't get your shit together and stick to your habits? Where will you be in ten years if you continue on the Fuckit trajectory? Thinking about this shit should hurt. If you are avoiding facing those yucky feelings, you are never going to have the Fucks to change your behavior.

But don't linger on the negative feelings and get all self-pitying. Remember that story when I was at acting school and we had to escape the room quietly in order to live? Those of us who focused on the pain of possibly dying...died. The one girl who focused on why she wanted to live was the only one who escaped the room and therefore lived. Once you've identified the painful consequences of buying real estate in Fuckittown, drop that vision entirely. Instead, redirect all your attention to the life you actually want. How would it feel if you were just as healthy and hot as you want to be? If your healthy habits felt like an effortless part of your identity? Where will you be in ten years if that change started to happen today? I bet it would feel pretty damn good. Which is the whole point. Feeling good. Happiness.

Once you've found your fucks, then...

STEP #3. REMEMBER THAT IT'S ALL ABOUT HAPPINESS NOW.

I know that the Fuckits can be a dark place. You are mad at yourself for breaking your intentions. You have a sneaking suspicion that you just don't have the strength of character necessary to do this shit. You might resent your stupid body for requiring the maintenance that it does. All these grumpy thoughts are totally natural. Remember that the

Fuckits are like puberty. You might feel like you want to lock yourself in your room because no one understands you and write bad poetry. I get it. (Just ask my tenth-grade English teacher. I should find that poor woman and send her thank-you flowers for taking seriously my 1992 epic poem, "Dark Shadows, Cast by the Moon.")

But now, with the benefit of maturity, we all know that kind of melodrama isn't particularly helpful. Remember that the ultimate goal here isn't really to eat vegetables or run a six-minute mile or even to lose weight and get smokin' hot. The ultimate goal is the *feeling* that you think you will have once you've accomplished those goals: happiness. And happiness will never come from marinating in yucky, self-hating, fuck-it thoughts.

Even though you might be mad at yourself, you have to forgive yourself and move on. Remember that it is impossible to "punish" yourself into good behavior. Self-punishing thoughts will lead to self-punishing behaviors. Bad feelings will lead to more bad feelings. This is exactly the opposite of what you want.

Self-punishing thoughts will lead to self-punishing behaviors. Bad feelings will lead to more bad feelings. This is exactly the opposite of what you want.

If you need help being gentle with yourself when you are in the Fuckits, picture yourself as a little baby who is learning to walk. You keep falling down on your little diaper bum, and you're getting frustrated and starting to cry. Would you get angry with that baby and yell at her because she isn't able to walk? Would that help? Would it result in her learning to walk faster? Of course not. What you would do is pick up the frustrated baby and comfort her and make her happy. Once she's happier, she is much more likely to have success. Frustrated babies are fucking useless. And so are you when you are in the Fuckit zone. So, your one job right now is to comfort your grumpy baby self. Go for a walk, call a funny friend, or do whatever you need to do to get out of your funk. I will often counsel my clients, after they've made regrettable choices: "This is not the end of the world. You are one workout away from feeling like yourself again."

Oh, by the way, when do you give up on the baby learning to walk? Never, obviously. Because walking rules. And you want the best life possible for your baby. Same goes for you and achieving exactly the body you choose. And this Healthy as Fuck habits-based approach *works*. You are on the right path. Making healthy habits part of your identity is the *only* way to long term health and hotness, and you now know exactly which keystone habits to focus on. Just because you are slightly off course right now doesn't mean that it's the wrong route for you or that the destination isn't worth it. If you keep coming home to your healthy habits and loving yourself every step of the way, you will be astounded by the change in your body and the quality of your one and only life on this planet. So when the Fuckits happen and you are having those yucky feelings, don't try to soothe yourself by getting distracted and tempted by the latest weight-loss fad. None of those fads work in the long run. You've probably already done that research, so don't waste your energetic resources doing it again, when you could be focusing on getting back on track with being the Healthy Motherfucker that you truly are.

If you need convincing that there is a light at the end of the Fuckit tunnel, there are all sorts of #fitspo before-and-after shots at www .fitfeelsgood.com/stories. But remember that the real transformation might look like this:

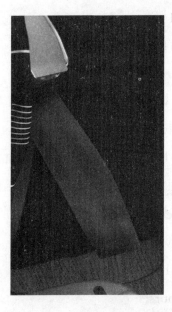

That's an airplane seat belt. My client Donna sent the photo to me because her healthy habits have resulted in a weight loss that meant she didn't have to ask for a seat-belt extender. And now that she doesn't have to face that humiliation, she wants to travel the world.

Or Evie, who always avoided getting in boats because she was afraid that she would be the one to tip it over. Here she is after her first day with the Dublin Dragon boating team:

Dragon boating, bitchaaaaaas! Did not fall on. Did not make a tit of myself!

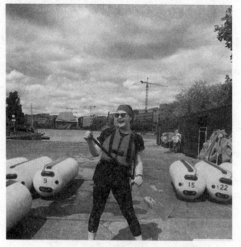

Or Rebecca, who was the classic sandwich generation woman: looking after parents and kids. She felt trapped by her circumstances and made her life smaller and smaller. The couch called to her after work, and she became less social as the weight piled on. She never wore anything other than black. She is shy, so she asked me to decapitate her in this before-and-after shot:

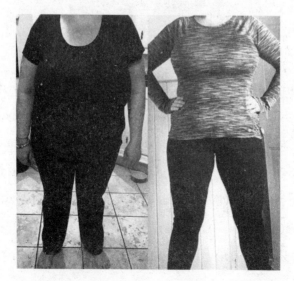

But she also said, "Tell them not to look at how much weight I've lost but how I *feel*. I am no longer waiting to live my damn *life*."

Starting to live your damn life can happen right now, at exactly the weight you are. Forgive your little baby self for getting the Fuckits, and proceed to step 4!

STEP #4. REVIEW YOUR KEYSTONE HABITS.

Let's review the 7 Habits of Highly Healthy Motherfuckers and get real about where you are being a slack-ass MOFO. Again, don't get all self-flagellant about it. This is just information that you can work with.

1. Are You Filling Half Your Plate with Vegetables?
   Wanna be part of the 1 percent? Then eat your damn vegetables. Research shows that there is a 99 percent chance you aren't getting the optimal ten servings of fruit and vegetables a day, which will automatically control your calorie intake and, um, help you not die.

2. Are You Getting at Least Seven Hours of Sleep?
   Since 1960, chronic sleep deprivation has increased dramatically in North America and—looky looky—so have our waistlines.

3. Do You Need to Take Another Step Back from the Booze?
   If you drink alcohol, you have to acknowledge that it sabotages

your fitness results, even if you are pristine in all your other habits. Is it time to back away from the booze?

4. **Do You Need to Practice a More Self-Loving Mindset or Chill the Fuck Out?**

Every time you start thinking of yourself as a fat fuck who has a cheese addiction, you will fulfill that prophecy. Drop the drama in your head using meditation and you will drop the extra junk around the middle.

5. **Do You Need to Rein In Your Portions?**

Remember that almost everyone who has excess body fat is just straight up eating too much. Period.

6. **Is It Time to Actually Prep and Plan in Advance?**

By now you've realized this shit doesn't just happen on its own. Dedicating an hour a week to meal prep is probably the most efficient use of your limited time if fat loss is your priority.

7. **Are You Exercising Consistently?**

No, you can't "work off" food. But exercising consistently is one of your strongest weapons against getting the Fuckits, and a key predictor of maintaining weight-loss results for the long term.

Have you identified your area of slackitude? Now that you know what's *not* working, let's get mega practical and figure this shit out.

STEP #5. IS THERE ANY WAY YOU COULD MAKE THIS HABIT EASIER?

Channel my dominatrix "get 'er done" former boss and ask yourself *How could I make this more fun and easy?* How could you set up your environment for success? Reduce distractions? Do you need to ask your friend for the name of her babysitter? What are the barriers getting in your way, and how can you hedge them off in advance? Could you take five minutes to automate reminders on your phone? Is it time for some kick-ass new music to get you pumped? Do you need to come up with a different bribe to make yourself actually want to do your habit? Often, the Fuckits are a result of life making your habits too hard. If that's the case, you might want to think about what needs to change in your life in order to support you being healthier and happier. Seriously. You've only got one life to live. Don't be a victim to your circumstances. Change what needs changing.

STEP #6. HOW COULD YOU RECRUIT MORE SOCIAL SUPPORT?

The best way to make something fun is to make it social. Even if you identify as an introvert, your peers will create the new normal you will conform to, for better or worse. So, is there any way you could make your healthy habit a group activity? Could you ask your family for more support? Is there a group that is already doing this shit so you can join it and learn from them? Don't be afraid to suck in front of other people. If you are dead serious about your new habit, grow a pair and make a public commitment so that your community can hold you accountable.

STEP #7. WHAT IS THE BULLSHIT YOU ARE USING TO GET OUT OF YOUR HABIT?

What was the thought that went through your head before you dove headfirst into the Fuckit pool?

Were you on vacation and decided to "pause" your habits because you were all like "YOLO, bitches!"?

Or maybe you were convincing yourself that while you'd really just love to be doing your habit, you unfortunately don't have time right now?

Rewind your mental tape to figure out what that clever brain of yours is coming up with in order to push you back to your comfort zone. It's just trying to protect you, but you are going to have to become consciously aware of it in order to politely decline. Come up with a break-up speech so that you don't fall for this seductive Bullshit again.

On the other hand, if your story about why you can't do your habit feels pretty legit, that's when you proceed to step 8!

STEP #8. HALF-ASS YOUR HABIT.

If your habits are collapsing faster than a game of Jenga with a toddler, you might be pushing yourself too hard, too fast. I get that you want results like, yesterday, but we are playing the long game here. That all-or-nothing, go-hard-or-go-home mentality is a recipe for a Fuckit soufflé. Instead of giving up, ask yourself: *What half-ass version of my habit could I realistically do* now *to start building that habit loop?*

Remember that those half-ass efforts totally count. One percent improvement every day doesn't sound that exciting until you see the glorious boner that is a compound-interest chart:

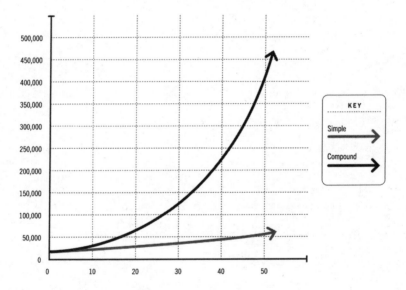

COMPOUND INTEREST

Now that's what I'm talking about. Those are the kind of results you can get from consistent, teeny-tiny improvements.

And remember, it's not that you are always perfect and never get the Fuckits. If that compound-interest chart were real life, it would be more of a jagged line with lots of ups and downs. All you have to do is make your highs a little higher and the lows also a little higher, and the Boner of Success will be yours.

So, shrug off the occasional bout of the Fuckits and focus on what you are doing right. And, dude. You are doing so much right.

CONCLUSION

YOU DID IT! I'M HERE AT THE FINISH LINE, JUMPING UP AND DOWN with excitement, ready to wrap you up in a medal and a big hug. I'm your coach looking at you with tears of pride right now. Wait, you think you haven't done anything yet?! You say you haven't yet laced up your running shoes, haven't even experimented with a green smoothie?

Maybe you think you haven't even started getting Healthy as Fuck—but you are wrong. In reading this book, you have already started to create a new identity: the identity of someone who chooses the life she wants and takes radical responsibility for creating it.

You are someone who has embraced your right to be just as healthy and hot as you want to be. Fuck anyone who makes you feel weird about your goals for your body.

You are someone who doesn't accept the cultural standard of being overweight, tired, and unhealthy. You accept that in order to get different results, you are going to have to do something different.

You are someone who has rejected the weight-loss media hype bullshit that steals your money and makes everyone feel like crap. You've excused yourself from the distractions of the next fad diet. You believe in the sanity of sustainable healthy habits. You aren't going to waste your efforts and emotions on silly fads because you know the seven simple yet profoundly effective habits that will give you an exceptional bod, unbelievable vitality, and a long and happy life.

You are no longer seduced by the Bullshit that wants to keep you in your comfort zone and hold you back. From now on you will always recognize those self-defeating thoughts as Bullshit, which means they have no power over you anymore.

You've dropped the all-or-nothing drama and celebrate every time you take even a tiny step toward your goals.

You are someone who never gives up on herself. Just like a baby learning to walk, you have endless patience, love, and total confidence that it's gonna happen for you—no matter how many times you fall down. You know that the falling down is part of the process. You just get back up with minimal drama and try again.

You have shown you are someone who is willing to do the real work of getting to know yourself, rather than spinning your wheels with the easy effort and busywork that never really changes anything.

Even if you read this whole book while munching on snacks and wearing your fuzzy slippers, you've already done a lot of that hard work of getting to know yourself as you read through these pages.

Most of all—you've come to realize that your life starts right *now*. Not when you reach your goal weight. Not even on Monday when you go for that first jog. Right now. As you read these words.

When you choose to be happy in this moment—exactly as you are—you are also loving yourself enough to know that you have unlimited potential.

Now close the book and get going with your new life. I'm proud of you, Motherfucker. X

NOTES

PREFACE

v   *1 percent of the population:* Choung, Rok Seon, Aynur Unalp-Arida, Constance E. Ruhl, Tricia L. Brantner, James E. Everhart, and Joseph A. Murray. "Less Hidden Celiac Disease but Increased Gluten Avoidance without a Diagnosis in the United States: Findings from the National Health and Nutrition Examination Surveys from 2009 to 2014." *Mayo Clinic Proceedings* 92, no. 1 (January 2017): 30–38. https://doi.org/10.1016/j.mayocp.2016.10.012.

vi   *actively trying to lose weight:* "Obesity in America: What Are the Consequences?" PublicHealth.org. Accessed November 6, 2018. https://www.publichealth.org/public-awareness/obesity/consequences.

vi   *30 percent of North Americans are clinically obese, 39.8% in the USA:* "Overweight & Obesity: Adult Obesity Facts." Centers for Disease Control and Prevention. Last modified August 13, 2018. https://www.cdc.gov/obesity/data/adult.html.

vi   *30 percent of North Americans are clinically obese, 27% in Canada:* Government of Canada. "Overweight and Obese Adults (self-reported), 2014." Statistics Canada. Updated November 27, 2015. https://www150.statcan.gc.ca/n1/pub/82-625-x/2015001/article /14185-eng.htm.

vi   *spending an average of $800 a year:* "Obesity in America: What Are the Consequences?" PublicHealth.org. Accessed November 6, 2018. https://www.publichealth.org/public-awareness/obesity /consequences.

vii   *better than any other for long-term weight loss:* Sacks, Frank M., George A. Bray, Vincent J. Carey, Steven R. Smith, Donna H. Ryan, Stephen D. Anton, Katherine McManus, et al. "Comparison of Weight-Loss Diets with Different Compositions of Fat, Protein, and Carbohydrates." *Obstetrical and Gynecological Survey* 64, no. 7 (July 2009): 460–62. https://doi.org/10.1097/01.ogx .0000351673.32059.13.

vii   *better than any other for long-term weight loss:* Gardner, Christopher D., John F. Trepanowski, Liana C. Del Gobbo, Michelle E. Hauser, Joseph Rigdon, John P. A. Ioannidis, Manisha Desai, and Abby C. King. "Effect of Low-Fat vs Low-Carbohydrate Diet on 12-Month Weight Loss in Overweight Adults and the Association with Genotype Pattern or Insulin Secretion: The DIETFITS Randomized Clinical Trial." *JAMA—Journal of the American Medical Association* 319, no. 7: 667–79. https://doi.org/10.1001/jama.2018.0245.

vii   *keeping the weight off for over a year:* Makoundou, V., F. Habicht, E. Bobbioni-Harsch, Z. Pataky, and A. Golay. "Long-Term Weight Loss Maintenance." *Revue Medicale Suisse* 6, no. 242 (March 2010): 682–84. https://doi.org/10.1093/ajcn/82.1.222S.

vii   *keeping the weight off for over a year:* Mann, Traci, A. Janet Tomiyama, Erika Westling, Ann-Marie Lew, Barbra Samuels, and Jason Chatman. "Medicare's Search for Effective Obesity Treatments: Diets Are Not the Answer." *American Psychologist* 62, no. 3 (April 2007): 220–33. https://doi.org/10.1037/0003-066X.62.3.220.

vii   *small changes to everyday behaviors:* Thomas, J. Graham, Dale S. Bond, Suzanne Phelan, James O. Hill, and Rena R. Wing. "Weight-Loss

Maintenance for 10 Years in the National Weight Control Registry."
American Journal of Preventive Medicine 46, no. 1 (January 2014):
17–23. https://doi.org/10.1016/j.amepre.2013.08.019.

PART 1
INTRODUCTION

3   *rising rates of obesity and type 2 diabetes in children:* "Obesity Update
        2017." Organisation for Economic Co-operation and Development.
        Accessed October 10, 2018. https://www.oecd.org/els/health-systems
        /Obesity-Update-2017.pdf.

Chapter 1

15   *talked about how obesity is socially constructed:* Hermiston, Alana
        J. "'Who are you calling "fat"?': The Social Construction of the
        Obesity Epidemic." Edited by Anaya Mukherjea. *Understanding
        Emerging Epidemics: Social and Political Approaches (Advances in
        Medical Sociology, Volume 11).* Emerald Group Publishing Limited,
        2010: 359–69. *For a quick primer on the subject, try:* Bias, Stacy.
        "Reclaiming Fat: Language, Social Constructs and Just Shaddup
        about It Already." *Stacy Bias—Heart-Led Creative* (blog). September
        14, 2010. http://stacybias.net/2010/09/reclaiming-fat-language-social
        -constructs-and-just-shaddup-about-it-already/.

16   *more than half of American women are trying to lose weight:* Martin,
        Crescent B., Kirsten A. Herrick, Neda Sarafrazi, and Cynthia L. Ogden.
        "Attempts to Lose Weight Among Adults in the United States, 2013–
        2016." Centers for Disease Control and Prevention. Updated July 12,
        2018. https://www.cdc.gov/nchs/products/databriefs/db313.htm.

Chapter 2

24   *It's a concept that's made the rounds in personal development circles:*
        Thompson, Geoff. "Difficult Difficult Difficult Easy." Inspire Daily.
        March 31, 2018. http://inspiredaily.co.uk/difficult-difficult-difficult
        -easy/.

24   *John Berardi of Precision Nutrition. Easy effort is hard work that feels familiar:* "Precision Nutrition." Facebook.com. October 26, 2015. https://www.facebook.com/insidePN/photos/a.133423386761301 /644672352303066/?type=1&theater.

Chapter 3

46   *A 2017 study from McGill University:* Duarte, Cristiana, Marcela Matos, R. James Stubbs, Corinne Gale, Liam Morris, Jose Pinto Gouveia, and Paul Gilbert. "The Impact of Shame, Self-Criticism and Social Rank on Eating Behaviours in Overweight and Obese Women Participating in a Weight Management Programme." *PLoS ONE* 12, no. 1 (January 2017). https://doi.org/10.1371/journal.pone.0167571.

46   *Another study done at Duke University:* Adams, Claire E., and Mark R. Leary. "Promoting Self-Compassionate Attitudes toward Eating Among Restrictive and Guilty Eaters." *Journal of Social and Clinical Psychology* 26, no. 10 (2007): 1120–44. https://doi.org/10.1521/jscp .2007.26.10.1120.

PART 2
INTRODUCTION

60   *Twenty-five percent of people abandon their New Year's resolutions after just one week:* Norcross, John C., Albert C. Ratzin, and Dorothy Payne. "Ringing in the New Year: The Change Processes and Reported Outcomes of Resolutions." *Addictive Behaviors* 14, no. 2 (1989): 205–12. https://doi.org/10.1016/0306-4603(89)90050-6.

60   *An overwhelming 60 percent of people have bailed on their resolution by February:* Norcross, John C., Albert C. Ratzin, and Dorothy Payne. "Ringing in the New Year: The Change Processes and Reported Outcomes of Resolutions." Addictive Behaviors 14, no. 2 (1989): 205–12. doi:10.1016/0306-4603(89)90050-6.

60   *The average person will make the same damn resolution five times without success:* Prochaska, James O., Carlo C. Diclemente, and John C. Norcross. "In Search of How People Change: Applications to

Addictive Behaviors." *Journal of Addictions Nursing* 5, no. 1 (January 1993): 2–16. https://doi.org/10.3109/10884609309149692.

60   *even after a heart attack, only 14 percent of patients make any lasting changes around eating or exercise:* Suaya, Jose A., Donald S. Shepard, Sharon-Lise T. Normand, Philip A. Ades, Jeffrey Prottas, and William B. Stason. "Use of Cardiac Rehabilitation by Medicare Beneficiaries after Myocardial Infarction or Coronary Bypass Surgery." *Circulation* 116, no. 15 (September 2007): 1653–62. https://doi.org/10.1161/CIRCULATIONAHA.107.701466.

63   *Madonna:* Bergland, Christopher. "The Neuroscience of Madonna's Enduring Success." *Psychology Today.* September 7, 2013. https://www.psychologytoday.com/ca/blog/the-athletes-way/201309/the-neuroscience-madonnas-enduring-success.

Chapter 4

67   *About 40 to 45 percent of our actions are habits we don't even think about:* Duhigg, Charles. *The Power of Habit: Why We Do What We Do in Life and Business.* New York: Random House, 2012.

Chapter 5

81   *filling half of every plate with vegetables:* Wang, Xia, Yingying Ouyang, Jun Liu, Minmin Zhu, Gang Zhao, Wei Bao, and Frank B. Hu. "Fruit and Vegetable Consumption and Mortality from All Causes, Cardiovascular Disease, and Cancer: Systematic Review and Dose-Response Meta-Analysis of Prospective Cohort Studies." *BMJ (Online)* 349 (July 2014). https://doi.org/10.1136/bmj.g4490.

84   *phytochemicals help prevent cardiovascular disease, cancer, type 2 diabetes, and age-related mental decline:* Webb, Densie. "Phytochemicals' Role in Good Health." *Today's Dietitian* 15, no. 9 (September 2013): 70. https://www.todaysdietitian.com/newarchives/090313p70.shtml.

85   *60 percent of Americans are now actively trying to increase their protein consumption:* Egan, Sophie. "How Much Protein Do We

Need?". Nytimes.com. July 28, 2017. https://www.nytimes.com/2017
/07/28/well/eat/how-much-protein-do-we-need.html.

85   *In Canada and the United States, the average person is consuming
      nearly twice as much protein as recommended:* Ranganathan, Janet.
      2016. "People Are Eating More Protein than They Need—Especially
      in Wealthy Regions." World Resources Institute. April 2016. https://
      www.wri.org/resources/charts-graphs/people-eating-more-protein
      -wealthy-regions.

86   *Consumers will spend more money on their food if the word* protein
      is emphasized: Bratskeir, Kate. "America's Obsession with Protein Is
      Just Another Silly Health Fad." Mic.com. September 9, 2016. https://
      mic.com/articles/153485/america-s-obsession-with-protein-is-just
      -another-silly-health-fad#.Vcz5dvK1Y

87   *Meta-analysis done by the Imperial College London:* Aune, Dagfinn,
      Edward Giovannucci, Paolo Boffetta, Lars T. Fadnes, NaNa Keum,
      Teresa Norat, Darren C. Greenwood, Elio Riboli, Lars J. Vatten,
      and Serena Tonstad. "Fruit and Vegetable Intake and the Risk of
      Cardiovascular Disease, Total Cancer and All-Cause Mortality—A
      Systematic Review and Dose-Response Meta-Analysis of Prospective
      Studies." *International Journal of Epidemiology* 46, no. 3 (June
      2017): 1029–56. https://doi.org/10.1093/ije/dyw319.

88   *0.83 grams of protein per kilo of body weight is sufficient for 97.5
      percent of the population:* World Health Organization. "Protein and
      Amino Acid Requirements in Human Nutrition: Report of a Joint
      WHO/FAO/UNU Expert Consultation." 2007. https://apps.who
      .int/iris/bitstream/handle/10665/43411/WHO_TRS_935_eng.pdf;
      jsessionid=A986615B15F458D0ED67606C78C07A26?sequence
      =1.

88   *the largest and most comprehensive study on human nutrition ever
      done:* Campbell, T. Colin, Thomas M. Campbell II. *The China Study:
      The most Comprehensive Study of Nutrition Ever Conducted and the
      Startling Implications for Diet, Weight Loss, and Long-Term Health.*
      Dallas: BenBella Books, 2006.

90   *Science says you are kidding yourself:* Williamson, A. M., and Anne-
        Marie Feyer. "Moderate Sleep Deprivation Produces Impairments in
        Cognitive and Motor Performance Equivalent to Legally Prescribed
        Levels of Alcohol Intoxication." *Occupational and Environmental
        Medicine* 57, no. 10 (October 2000): 649–55. https://doi.org/10.1136
        /oem.57.10.649.

90   *Everyone needs at least seven hours of sleep a night in order to
        function optimally:* Watson, Nathaniel F., M. Safwan Badr, Gregory
        Belenky, Donald L. Bliwise, Orfeu M. Buxton, Daniel Buysse, David
        F. Dinges, et al. "Joint Consensus Statement of the American Academy
        of Sleep Medicine and Sleep Research Society on the Recommended
        Amount of Sleep for a Healthy Adult: Methodology and Discussion."
        Journal of Clinical Sleep Medicine 11, no. 8 (2015): 931–52. https://
        doi.org/10.5664/jcsm.4950.

90   *Lack of sleep produces cortisol:* Wright, Kenneth P., Jr., Amanda L.
        Drake, Danielle J. Frey, Monika Fleshner, Christopher A. Desouza,
        Claude Gronfier, and Charles A. Czeisler. "Influence of Sleep
        Deprivation and Circadian Misalignment on Cortisol, Inflammatory
        Markers, and Cytokine Balance." *Brain, Behavior, and Immunity* 47
        (July 2015): 24–34. https://doi.org/10.1016/j.bbi.2015.01.004.

91   *Deep sleep releases growth hormone:* Van Cauter, Eve, and Laurence
        Plat. "Physiology of Growth Hormone Secretion during Sleep." *The
        Journal of Pediatrics* 128, no. 5 (May 1996): S32–37. https://doi.org
        /10.1016/S0022–3476(96)70008–2.

91   *ghrelin, leptin, insulin:* Donga, Esther, Marieke van Dijk, J. Gert
        van Dijk, Nienke R. Biermasz, Gert-Jan Lammers, Klaas W. van
        Kralingen, Eleonara P. M. Corssmit, and Johannes A. Romijn. "A
        Single Night of Partial Sleep Deprivation Induces Insulin Resistance
        in Multiple Metabolic Pathways in Healthy Subjects." *Journal of
        Clinical Endocrinology and Metabolism* 95, no. 6 (June 2010): 2963–
        68. https://doi.org/10.1210/jc.2009–2430.

91   *ghrelin, leptin, insulin:* Wang, Xuewen, Julian Greer, Ryan R. Porter,
        Kamaljeet Kaur, and Shawn D. Youngstedt. "Short-Term Moderate

Sleep Restriction Decreases Insulin Sensitivity in Young Healthy Adults." *Sleep Health* 2, no. 1 (March 2016): 63–68. https://doi.org /10.1016/j.sleh.2015.11.004.

91   *ghrelin, leptin, insulin:* Morselli, Lisa, Rachel Leproult, Marcella Balbo, and Karine Spiegel. "Role of Sleep Duration in the Regulation of Glucose Metabolism and Appetite." *Best Practice and Research: Clinical Endocrinology and Metabolism* 24, no. 5 (October 2010): 687–702. https://doi.org/10.1016/j.beem.2010.07.005.

92   *A lack of sleep can make you prone to getting colds and the flu:* Majde, Jeannine A., and James M. Krueger. "Links between the Innate Immune System and Sleep." *Journal of Allergy and Clinical Immunology* 116, no. 6 (December 2005): 1188–98. https://doi.org /10.1016/j.jaci.2005.08.005.

92   *A lack of sleep can make you prone to getting colds and the flu:* Cohen, Sheldon, William J. Doyle, Cuneyt M. Alper, Denise Janicki-Deverts, and Ronald B. Turner. "Sleep Habits and Susceptibility to the Common Cold." *Arch Intern Med* 169, no. 1 (January 2009): 62–67. https://doi.org/10.1001/archinternmed.2008.505.

93   *exercise at any time of day will promote a better sleep than not exercising at all:* Yang, Pei-Yu, Ka-Hou Ho, Hsi-Chung Chen, and Meng-Yueh Chien. "Exercise Training Improves Sleep Quality in Middle-Aged and Older Adults with Sleep Problems: A Systematic Review." *Journal of Physiotherapy* 58, no. 3 (September 2012): 157–63. https://doi.org/10.1016/S1836–9553(12)70106–6.

93   *magnesium helps you sleep:* Abbasi, Behnood, Masud Kimiagar, Khosro Sadeghniiat, Minoo M. Shirazi, Mehdi Hedayati, and Bahram Rashidkhani. "The Effect of Magnesium Supplementation on Primary Insomnia in Elderly: A Double-Blind Placebo-Controlled Clinical Trial." *Journal of Research in Medical Sciences* 17, no. 12 (December 2012): 1161–69. https://www.ncbi.nlm.nih.gov/pmc /articles/PMC3703169/.

94   *exposure to sunlight can help regulate circadian rhythms:* Dodson, Ehren R., and Phyllis C. Zee. "Therapeutics for Circadian Rhythm

Sleep Disorders." *Sleep Medicine Clinics* 5, no. 4 (December 2010): 701–15. https://doi.org/10.1016/j.jsmc.2010.08.001.

94   *wine and sleep:* Colrain, Ian M., Christian L. Nicholas, and Fiona C. Baker. "Alcohol and the Sleeping Brain." *Handbook of Clinical Neurology* 125 (2014): 415–31. https://doi.org/10.1016/B978-0 -444-62619-6.00024-0.

94   *wine and sleep:* Ebrahim, Irshaad O., Colin M. Shapiro, Adrian J. Williams, and Peter B. Fenwick. "Alcohol and Sleep I: Effects on Normal Sleep." *Alcoholism: Clinical and Experimental Research* 37, no. 4 (January 2013): 539–49. https://doi.org/10.1111/acer.12006.

95   *No amount of alcohol has been proven to be safe:* Griswold, Max G., Nancy Fullman, Caitlin Hawley, Nicholas Arian, Stephanie R. M. Zimsen, Hayley D. Tymeson, and Vidhya Venkateswaran, et al. "Alcohol Use and Burden for 195 Countries and Territories, 1990– 2016: A Systematic Analysis for the Global Burden of Disease Study 2016." *Lancet* 392, no. 10152 (September 2018): 1015–35. https:// doi.org/10.1016/s0140–6736(18)31310–2.

96   *drinking guidelines:* Office of Disease Prevention and Health Promotion. "United States Dietary Guidelines (2015–2020). Appendix 9: Alcohol." Accessed January 5, 2018. https://health.gov /dietaryguidelines/2015/guidelines/appendix-9/#table-a9–1.

97   *alcohol use in women in the developed world has skyrocketed over the past decade:* Johnston, Ann Dowsett. *Drink: The Intimate Relationship between Women and Alcohol.* New York: HarperCollins, 2013.

98   *a third of alcohol-related cancer deaths among women were associated with less than two standard drinks per day:* Kindy, Kimberly, and Dan Keating. "For Women, Heavy Drinking Has Been Normalized. That's Dangerous." *Washington Post.* December 13, 2016. https:// www.washingtonpost.com/national/for-women-heavy-drinking -has-been-normalized-thats-dangerous/2016/12/23/0e701120-c381 -11e6-9578-0054287507db_story.html?utm_term=.f0a38201f996.

98   *moderate drinkers have the lowest risk of early mortality:* Ellison, R.

Curtis. "Update on the J-Shaped Curve for the Relation of Alcohol Intake to Health." *Aim Digest*. Updated March 8, 2017. http://www.aim-digest.com/gateway/pages/moderate/articles/j-shaped_curve1.htm.

100   *"The current and emerging science does not support the purported benefits of moderate drinking"*: Kindy, Kimberly. "Heavy drinking has been normalized for women, and it's killing them in record numbers." *The Star*. December 23, 2016. https://www.thestar.com/news/world/2016/12/23/heavy-drinking-has-been-normalized-for-women-and-its-killing-them-in-record-numbers.html.

106   *acute "what doesn't kill you makes you stronger" stress*: Tonhajzerova, I., and M. Mestanik. "New Perspectives in the Model of Stress Response." *Physiological Research* 66, suppl. 2 (2017): S173-S185. http://www.biomed.cas.cz/physiolres/pdf/66/66_S173.pdf.

106   *chronic stress...increases our risk of heart disease*: Tonhajzerova, I., and M. Mestanik. "New Perspectives in the Model of Stress Response." *Physiological Research* 66, suppl. 2 (2017): S173-S185. http://www.biomed.cas.cz/physiolres/pdf/66/66_S173.pdf.

107   *Chronic stress leads to anxiety, depression, and sleep disorders, and then it increases our appetites and makes us crave sugar and fat*: Epel, Elissa, Rachel Lapidus, Bruce McEwen, and Kelly Brownell. "Stress May Add Bite to Appetite in Women: A Laboratory Study of Stress-Induced Cortisol and Eating Behavior." *Psychoneuroendocrinology* 26, no. 1 (January 2001): 37–49. https://doi.org/10.1016/S0306-4530(00)00035-4.

111   *meditation...can reduce the inflammation caused by stress, decrease your blood pressure, help you sleep, reduce chronic pain, and improve your emotional health in almost every way*: Thorpe, Matthew. "12 Science-Based Benefits of Meditation." *Healthline*. July 5, 2017. https://www.healthline.com/nutrition/12-benefits-of-meditation.

111   *meditation will decrease activity in the amygdala*: Hölzel, Britta K., James Carmody, Karleyton C. Evans, Elizabeth A. Hoge, Jeffery A.

Dusek, Lucas Morgan, Roger K. Pitman, and Sara W. Lazar. "Stress Reduction Correlates with Structural Changes in the Amygdala." *Social Cognitive and Affective Neuroscience* 5, no. 1 (March 2010): 11–17. https://doi.org/10.1093/scan/nsp034.

112   *meditation…strengthens areas of the brain that are involved in emotional regulation, body awareness, and introspection:* Fox, Kieran C. R., Savannah Nijeboer, Matthew L. Dixon, James L. Floman, Melissa Ellamil, Samuel P. Rumak, Peter Sedlmeier, and Kalina Christoff. "Is Meditation Associated with Altered Brain Structure? A Systematic Review and Meta-Analysis of Morphometric Neuroimaging in Meditation Practitioners." *Neuroscience and Biobehavioral Reviews* 43 (June 2014): 48–73. https://doi.org/10.1016/j.neubiorev.2014 .03.016.

116   *when given low-fat foods, subjects will consume 60 percent more calories:* Wansink, Brian, and Pierre Chandon. "Can 'Low-Fat' Nutrition Labels Lead to Obesity?" *Journal of Marketing Research* 43, no. 4 (November 2006): 605–17. https://doi.org/10.1509/jmkr.43.4.605.

116   *protein:* Anderson, G. Harvey, and Shannon E. Moore. "The Emerging Role of Dairy Proteins and Bioactive Peptides in Nutrition and Health: Dietary Proteins in the Regulation of Food Intake and Body Weight in Humans." *Journal of Nutrition* 134, no. 4 (2004): 974–79. http://veggieprotein.com.br/artigos/neutro/7.pdf.

116   *protein:* Halton, Thomas L., and Frank B. Hu. "The Effects of High Protein Diets on Thermogenesis, Satiety and Weight Loss: A Critical Review." *Journal of the American College of Nutrition* 23, no. 5 (2004): 373–85. https://doi.org/10.1080/07315724.2004.10719381.

116   *protein:* Westerterp-Plantenga, M.S., A. Nieuwenhuizen, D. Tomé, S. Soenen, and K. R. Westerterp. "Dietary Protein, Weight Loss, and Weight Maintenance." *Annual Review of Nutrition* 29, no. 1 (August 2009): 21–41. https://doi.org/10.1146/annurev-nutr-080508-141056.

117   *seriously avoid processed meat and deli slices and fatty meat like bacon:* Larsson, Susanna C., and Nicola Orsini. "Red Meat and Processed Meat Consumption and All-Cause Mortality: A Meta-Analysis."

American Journal of Epidemiology 179, no. 3 (February 2014): 282–89. https://doi.org/10.1093/aje/kwt261.

117 *seriously avoid processed meat and deli slices and fatty meat like bacon:* Wang, Xia, Xinying Lin, Ying Y. Ouyang, Jun Liu, Gang Zhao, An Pan, and Frank B. Hu. "Red and Processed Meat Consumption and Mortality: Dose-Response Meta-Analysis of Prospective Cohort Studies." *Public Health Nutrition* 19, no. 5 (April 2016): 893–905. https://doi.org/10.1017/S1368980015002062.

117 *seriously avoid processed meat and deli slices and fatty meat like bacon:* Richi, Evelyne Battaglia, Beatrice Baumer, Beatrice Conrad, Roger Darioli, Alexandra Schmid, and Ulrich Keller. "Health Risks Associated with Meat Consumption: A Review of Epidemiological Studies." *International Journal for Vitamin and Nutrition Research* 85 (2015): 70–78. https://doi.org/10.1024/0300-9831/a000224.

117 *seriously avoid processed meat and deli slices and fatty meat like bacon:* Abete, Itziar, Dora Romaguera, Ana Rita Vieira, Adolfo Lopez de Munain, and Teresa Norat. "Association between Total, Processed, Red and White Meat Consumption and All-Cause, CVD and IHD Mortality: A Meta-Analysis of Cohort Studies." *British Journal of Nutrition* 112, no. 5 (September 2014): 762–75. https://doi.org/10.1017/S000711451400124X.

119 *The WHO recommends that sugar account for no more than 5 percent of our caloric intake:* "Guideline: Sugars Intake for Adults and Children." World Health Organization, 2015. Accessed January 5, 2018. http://apps.who.int/iris/bitstream/handle/10665/149782/9789241549028_eng.pdf?sequence=1.

119 *The average North American gets three times that amount each day:* Welsh, Jean A., Andrea J. Sharma, Lisa Grellinger, and Miriam B. Vos. "Consumption of Added Sugars Is Decreasing in the United States." *American Journal of Clinical Nutrition* 94, no. 3 (September 2011): 726–34. https://doi.org/10.3945/ajcn.111.018366.

121 *even a 2 percent increase of calories from trans fats has been associated with a 34 percent increase in all-cause mortality:* de Souza,

Russell J., Andrew Mente, Adriana Maroleanu, Adrian I. Cozma, Vanessa Ha, Teruko Kishibe, Elizabeth Uleryk, et al. "Intake of Saturated and Trans Unsaturated Fatty Acids and Risk of All Cause Mortality, Cardiovascular Disease, and Type 2 Diabetes: Systematic Review and Meta-Analysis of Observational Studies." *BMJ (Online)* 351 (August 2015). https://doi.org/10.1136/bmj.h3978.

134   *the same fat-burning results with less time spent exercising:* Hazell, Tom J., T. Dylan Olver, Craig D. Hamilton, and Peter W. R. Lemon. "Two Minutes of Sprint-Interval Exercise Elicits 24-Hr Oxygen Consumption Similar to That of 30 Min of Continuous Endurance Exercise." *International Journal of Sport Nutrition and Exercise Metabolism* 22, no. 4 (June 2012): 276–83. https://doi.org/10.1123/ijsnem.22.4.276.

134   *the same fat-burning results with less time spent exercising:* Skelly, Lauren E., Patricia C. Andrews, Jenna B. Gillen, Brian J. Martin, Michael E. Percival, and Martin J. Gibala. "High-Intensity Interval Exercise Induces 24-H Energy Expenditure Similar to Traditional Endurance Exercise despite Reduced Time Commitment." *Applied Physiology, Nutrition, and Metabolism* 39, no. 7 (2014): 845–48. https://doi.org/10.1139/apnm-2013-1340562.

141   *most North Americans get only about five thousand steps a day:* Bassett, David R., Holly R. Wyatt, Helen Thompson, John C. Peters, and James O. Hill. "Pedometer-Measured Physical Activity and Health Behaviors in U.S. Adults." *Medicine and Science in Sports and Exercise* 42, no. 10 (October 2010): 1819–25. https://doi.org/10.1249/MSS.0b013e3181dc2e54.

143   *NEAT is one of the most underrated components of wellness:* Levine, James A. "Non-Exercise Activity Thermogenesis (NEAT)." *Best Practice and Research: Clinical Endocrinology and Metabolism* 16, no. 4 (2002): 679–702. https://doi.org/10.1053/beem.2002.0227.

143   *Sleep better:* Van Cauter, Eve, and Laurence Plat. 1996. "Physiology of Growth Hormone Secretion during Sleep." *The Journal of Pediatrics* 128 (5): S32–37. https://www.jpeds.com/article/S0022-3476(96)70008-2/fulltext.

143   *Reduce the risk of dementia:* Hyodo, Kazuki, Ippeita Dan, Yasushi
       Kyutoku, Kazuya Suwabe, Kyeongho Byun, Genta Ochi, Morimasa
       Kato, and Hideaki Soya. "The Association between Aerobic Fitness and
       Cognitive Function in Older Men Mediated by Frontal Lateralization."
       NeuroImage 125 (January 2016): 291–300. https://doi.org/10.1016
       /j.neuroimage.2015.09.062.

143   *Improve your bone strength:* "Fact Sheet: Physical Activity." World
       Health Organization. February 23, 2018. http://www.who.int/news
       -room/fact-sheets/detail/physical-activity.

144   *Have better sex:* Lane-Cordova, Abbi D., Kiarri Kershaw, Kiang Liu,
       David Herrington, and Donald M. Lloyd-Jones. "Association between
       Cardiovascular Health and Endothelial Function with Future Erectile
       Dysfunction: The Multi-Ethnic Study of Atherosclerosis." *American
       Journal of Hypertension* 30, no. 8 (August 2017): 815–21. https://doi
       .org/10.1093/ajh/hpx060.

144   *Reduce depression:* Kvam, Siri, Catrine Lykkedrang Kleppe, Inger
       Hilde Nordhus, and Anders Hovland. "Exercise as a Treatment for
       Depression: A Meta-Analysis." *Journal of Affective Disorders* 202
       (September 2016): 67–86. https://doi.org/10.1016/j.jad.2016.03.063.

144   *When you increase your lean muscle mass, you will have an elevated
       resting metabolism:* Zurlo, Francesco, Karen Larson, Clifton
       Bogardus, and Eric Ravussin. "Skeletal Muscle Metabolism Is a Major
       Determinant of Resting Energy Expenditure." *Journal of Clinical
       Investigation* 86, no. 5 (November 1990): 1423–27. https://doi.org
       /10.1172/JCI114857.

145   *the most effective training program for belly fat reduction for older
       adults was strength training for twenty minutes a day along with
       aerobic training:* Mekary, Rania A., Anders Grøntved, Jean-Pierre
       Despres, Leandro Pereira De Moura, Morteza Asgarzadeh, Walter
       C. Willett, Eric B. Rimm, Edward Giovannucci, and Frank B. Hu.
       "Weight Training, Aerobic Physical Activities, and Long-Term Waist
       Circumference Change in Men." *Obesity* 23, no. 2 (February 2015):
       461–67. https://doi.org/10.1002/oby.20949.

145   *HIIT and strength training:* Heden, Timothy, Curt Lox, Paul Rose, Steven Reid, and Erik P. Kirk. "One-Set Resistance Training Elevates Energy Expenditure for 72 H Similar to Three Sets." *European Journal of Applied Physiology* 111, no. 3 (March 2011): 477–84. https://doi.org/10.1007/s00421-010-1666-5.

145   *HIIT and strength training:* Greer, Beau Kjerulf, Prawee Sirithienthad, Robert J. Moffatt, Richard T. Marcello, and Lynn B. Panton. "EPOC Comparison between Isocaloric Bouts of Steady-State Aerobic, Intermittent Aerobic, and Resistance Training." *Research Quarterly for Exercise and Sport* 86, no. 2 (2015): 190–95. https://doi.org/10.1080 /02701367.2014.999190.

146   *natural exercise-induced endorphins:* Mikkelsen, Kathleen, Lily Stojanovska, Momir Polenakovic, Marijan Bosevski, and Vasso Apostolopoulos. "Exercise and Mental Health." *Maturitas* 106 (December 2017): 48–56. https://doi.org/10.1016/j.maturitas.2017.09 .003.

PART 3
Chapter 7

175   *Obese or overweight (60 percent of North Americans):* Murray, Christopher J. L., Marie Ng, and Ali Mokdad. "The Vast Majority of American Adults Are Overweight or Obese, and Weight Is a Growing Problem among US Children." Institute for Health Metrics and Evaluation. May 28, 2014. http://www.healthdata.org/news-release /vast-majority-american-adults-are-overweight-or-obese-and-weight -growing-problem-among.

175   *Stressed (77 percent of Americans):* American Psychological Association. "Stress in America: Paying with Our Health." February 4, 2015. https:// www.apa.org/news/press/releases/stress/2014/stress-report.pdf.

175   *In debt (49 percent of Americans):* Tsosie, Claire, and Erin El Issa. "2018 American Household Credit Card Debt Study." NerdWallet. December 10, 2018. http://www.nerdwallet.com/blog/average-credit -card-debt-household/.

175   *Underslept (35.3 percent of Americans):* McKnight-Eily, L. R., Y. Liu, A. G. Wheaton, J. B. Croft, G. S. Perry, C. A. Okoro, and T. Strine. "Unhealthy Sleep-Related Behaviors—12 States, 2009." *Morbidity and Mortality Weekly Report (MMWR)* 60, no. 8 (March 2011): 233–38. https://www.cdc.gov/mmwr/preview/mmwrhtml/mm6008a2.htm.

175   *Binge drinking at least once a month (26 percent of Americans):* Dawson, Deborah A., Rise B. Goldstein, Tulshi D. Saha, and Bridget F. Grant. "Changes in Alcohol Consumption: United States, 2001–2002 to 2012–2013." *Drug and Alcohol Dependence* 148 (March 2015): 56–61. https://doi.org/10.1016/j.drugalcdep.2014.12.016.

175   *Not moving nearly enough to be healthy (80 percent of Americans):* Division of Nutrition, Physical Activity, and Obesity at the National Center for Chronic Disease Prevention and Health Promotion. Data, Trend, and Maps [online]. Centers for Disease Control and Prevention. Last modified September 27, 2018. https://www.cdc.gov/nccdphp/dnpao/data-trends-maps/index.html.

176   *Sensing social disapproval can actually trigger our brain's danger systems:* Eisenberger, Naomi I. "The Neural Bases of Social Pain: Evidence for Shared Representations with Physical Pain." *Psychosomatic Medicine* 74, no. 2 (February 2012): 126–35. https://doi.org/10.1097/PSY.0b013e3182464dd1.

176   *1950s study by Solomon Asch:* Asch, Solomon E. "Studies of Independence and Conformity: I. A Minority of One against a Unanimous Majority." *Psychological Monographs: General and Applied* 70, no. 9 (1956): 1–70. https://doi.org/10.1037/h0093718.

178   *online weight-loss communities can play a prominent role in weight-loss success:* Hwang, Kevin O., Allison J. Ottenbacher, Angela P. Green, M. Roseann Cannon-Diehl, Oneka Richardson, Elmer V. Bernstam, and Eric J. Thomas. "Social Support in an Internet Weight Loss Community." *International Journal of Medical Informatics* 79, no. 1 (January 2010): 5–13. https://doi.org/10.1016/j.ijmedinf.2009.10.003.

180   *75 percent of women "rarely or never" got support from friends or family in their weight-loss efforts:* Kiernan, Michaela, Susan D. Moore, Danielle E. Schoffman, Katherine Lee, Abby C. King, C. Barr Taylor, Nancy E. Kiernan, and Michael G. Perri. "Social Support for Healthy Behaviors: Scale Psychometrics and Prediction of Weight Loss among Women in a Behavioral Program." *Obesity* 20, no. 4 (April 2012): 756–64. https://doi.org/10.1038/oby.2011.293.

181   *sabotage friends' weight-loss efforts:* Perry, Keith. "Friends Are a Fat Lot of Good If You Are Trying to Lose Weight." *Telegraph.* January 9, 2014. https://www.telegraph.co.uk/lifestyle/wellbeing/diet/10562343 /Friends-are-a-fat-lot-of-good-if-you-are-trying-to-lose-weight.html.

Chapter 10

239   *you aren't getting the optimal ten servings of fruit and vegetables a day:* "The Changing American Diet: A Report Card." Center for Science in the Public Interest. September 23, 2013. https://cspinet.org/resource /changing-american-diet.

239   *chronic sleep deprivation has increased dramatically in North America:* Centers for Disease Control and Prevention. "Percentage of Adults Who Reported an Average of <6 Hours of Sleep per 24-Hour Period, by Sex and Age Group—United States, 1985 and 2004." *Morbidity and Mortality Weekly Report.* 2005. https://www.cdc.gov/mmwr/preview /mmwrhtml/mm5437a7.htm.

ACKNOWLEDGMENTS

All my gratitude goes first and foremost to my husband, Dylan, who delivered countless beautifully garnished salads to me at my computer, gave me shoulder rubs, and whisked our boys away on grocery shopping adventures so I could get work done. Basically, Dylan has done for me the unseen work that women have done for generations so that men could shine in their careers, and I would be a total dickhead not to acknowledge that I've benefited greatly from all that support—and I pretty much get all the limelight for myself. Dyl, this book (and much of the best parts of my life) wouldn't exist without you. You've always done way more than your share behind the scenes, and I'm so grateful. Thank you for bringing so much fun and silliness into our family and being such a wonderful husband to me and dad to the boys. I love you, and I'm so lucky to have you.

To Felix and Buddy: You little beasties are the light and joy of my days. Thank you for being so understanding when I was working so much and not being very fun. Instead of making me feel guilty, you would make very grown-up dinner conversation by asking me how my book was coming along. I'm so proud to have such interesting, supportive, and loving boys. I love you both to the moon and back, times infinity.

I also need to acknowledge early supporters of this book, starting with Denise Hendlarski, who set all the wheels in motion when she shrugged at my Bullshit when I told her that I would love to write a book but I didn't have time. Denise, thank you so much for challenging me to a higher standard, for the writing dates in weird co-working spaces, and for reading early versions of my work when I *know* you didn't have the time either. I can't wait for your book to come out.

To Ann Sheybani, who is the content editor genius who helped me put together a proposal that got attention for a totally unknown writer. Ann, thank you for encouraging me to just get this done by telling me to send you "total cat shit" and sifting through it for gold. I'm so grateful that our paths aligned.

To Sarah Lazarovic and Ben Erret, who answered a million questions about writing books, made it seem like no big whoop (because they are the kind of people who just do awesome stuff all the time), and put their rep on the line by connecting their fitness instructor friend with their agents and publishing contacts. Tanya Tagaq, you hooked me up large as well. Thank you, girl.

To Shanny, who will always be my most trusted sounding board for all of my projects—and my best friend. To James, who was so happy for me like only a true booklover could be.

To my agent, Sam Hiyate: Sam, I can't believe I thought I might just try to do this book stuff without an agent. That would have been so stupid. So grateful to have found the perfect one for me and so grateful for all your support and enthusiasm for this book.

To the Fit Feels Good Bootcampers and The Merkin Wolfpack: Thank you for being the best crew and making my job so much fun. You inspired me every day with your sweat, determination, and creative use of profanity when doing a burpee Tabata. Camille, thank you for calling me out of retirement; otherwise, none of this would have happened.

To my Transformers, and especially the MFers: This book was intended as a love letter to you. I can't tell you how profoundly affected I have been to witness your healthy journeys, your triumphs, your resilience, and the love and support you give each other. Not to mention the fact that you often do it all while being fucking hilarious. It is an honor to lead you, and I love you guys so much.

To Meesh, Jess, and Dyl: Thank you for basically running my company while I disappeared into a book hole—and for caring for our clients and our mission as much as I do.

Thank you to early readers like Bruce Mylrea, who offered his time, support, and valuable research skills to a total stranger because he's so passionate about healthy living. To Nadia Pestrak, who did the final polish to my proposal and sent spontaneous texts of excitement and support for the project. To dietitian Tricia Silverman, a presenter at a fitness conference who encouraged me to try out for Midwest Fitness Idol and then double-checked all my nutrition claims in this book. To Terri Brunsting, who set the first eyes on my chapter drafts and was so enthusiastic and awesome that she gave me the confidence to push forward to the next. To Sara Thompson, whose invaluable research skills have helped me not make a total ass of myself by triple-checking that all my sciencey smack talk in this book is legit.

To Dad and Cathy, Mum and Jim, and my lovely in-laws Don and Sandy Laister, who always swoop in with child care and home-cooked meals exactly when Dylan and I need it most.

To my editors: Laura Dosky at Penguin and Shana Drehs at Sourcebooks. I can't tell you how grateful I am to both of you for taking on this project and being so enthusiastic about it from the very beginning. It's a way better book because I had the benefit of your brains on it.

To Jeff Walker, my Durango Mastermind and Launch Club for all the support and coaching…but, most of all, for expanding my horizons of what is possible.

And finally, if I can be so cheeky as to sneak in another dedication before you start playing the Academy Awards get-off-the-damn-stage music in your head—I want to acknowledge my totally awesome grandmother, Oonagh McNerney, who died as I was finishing the final draft of this book. Mamon was wonderful and inspiring and so funny. She encouraged everyone around her (from her grandchildren to surprised strangers in an elevator) to "Be happy. Look lovely. Take care of yourself." This book is my long-winded way of passing on that awesome advice to you—and sending it with tons of love.

Oonagh x

ABOUT THE AUTHOR

Oonagh Duncan is a multiaward-winning fitness expert, author, and speaker specializing in helping women get lean, strong, and healthy through a habits-based approach. Her unique formula has resulted in international media attention, speaking engagements on stages in front of thousands, and, most importantly, five-star reviews from the thousands of people who have changed their lives through her programs.

Oonagh is the founder of the Feel Good Movement, which recognizes that fitness is not about a number on the scale but about feeling good. Because if you want to reach your highest potential and generally kick ass at life, it starts with feeling good *right now*. To feel good, Oonagh likes green smoothies and guilty pleasure '90s hip-hop dance parties with her family in the kitchen.